NEUROENDOCRINE TUMOR

Edited by **Anthony Lowell**

Neuroendocrine Tumor
Edited by Anthony Lowell

Published by InTech
Janeza Trdine 9, 51000 Rijeka, Croatia

Publishing Process Manager Dragana Manestar

Technical Editor Teodora Smiljanic

Cover Designer InTech Design Team

Additional hard copies can be obtained from orders@intechopen.com

Neuroendocrine Tumor, Edited by Anthony Lowell
p. cm.
ISBN 978-953-51-0653-1

For EU product safety concerns:
IN TECH d.o.o., Prolaz Marije Krucifikse Kozulić 3, 51000 Rijeka, Croatia,
info@intechopen.com or visit our website at intechopen.com.

Contents

1

The Association of Chronic Inflammation and Gastroenteropancreatic Neuroendocrine Tumors (GEP-NETs)

Maja Cigrovski Berković[1], Davorka Herman Mahečić[1], Vedran Tomašić[2], Davor Hrabar[2] and Vanja Zjačić-Rotkvić[1]

[1]*Department of Endocrinology, Diabetes and Metabolism University Hospital Centre "Sestre milosrdnice", Zagreb,*

[2]*Department of Gastroenterology and Hepathology University Hospital Centre "Sestre milosrdnice", Zagreb,*

Croatia

1. Introduction

Gastroenteropancreatic neuroendocrine tumors (GEP-NETs) are rare and heterogeneous neoplasms with overall increasing incidence, but not an associated increase in survival rate over the past few decades. Tumors originate from at least 16 different cells of diffuse endocrine system (DES), scattered through mucosa of gastrointestinal tract. They are mainly sporadic, but sometimes exhibit familial inheritance. Tumors often preserve the ability to synthesize, store and secrete numerous hormones and biogenic amines which sometimes lead to distinct hypersecretory and clinically recognizable syndromes (such as carcinoid, Zollinger-Ellison, WDHA etc.).[1] The resulting clinical symptoms are generally well controlled by somatostatin analogs and/or interferon-α.[2]

More often, GEP-NETs remain clinically silent until late, when they present with mass effect, and have unfortunately already locally or distantly spread. In the later case tumor growth and spread are not always well controlled by either biotherapy or chemotherapy. Although many biochemical and tissue markers for GEP-NETs already exist, sensitive and specific markers that predict tumor growth and behavior are lacking.[3]

According to our unpublished data chromogranin A (CgA) and 5-hydroxyindolacetic acid (5-HIAA), currently used as standard biochemical markers of neuroendocrine tumors were only positive in 76.84% and 20.79% of GEP-NET cases respectively. Tumor markers were analyzed in 101 patients (61.2% with localized and 38.8% with metastatic disease) diagnosed with GEP-NETs. According to same investigation, CgA levels were much higher when tumors were part of MEN1 syndrome, while 5-HIAA levels were higher in case of metastatic disease, especially when hepatic metastases were present. When 5-HIAA values were compared among patients with different tumor localizations, the highest values were detected in patients with functional midgut tumors. This is consistent with data of other authors on biochemical diagnostics of gastrointestinal neuroendocrine tumors.[4]

Unfortunately, the correct diagnose of GEP-NETs is delayed for 7-10 years, additionally adding burden to anyhow complex and challenging tumor management.[3] So, in clinical practice, more reliable serum markers as well as precise tumor localization of small, initial lesions together with incorporation of a histological grading system with implemented prognostic implications would help in optimal treatment of patients. The mentioned needs to be supported by better understanding of tumor cell biology and mechanistic regulation of underlying growth processes.[5]

In general, majority of GEP-NETs are represented by well-differentiated cells, and one would expect low proliferating rate, but unfortunately, tumors often present metastatic at the time of diagnosis. This is one of the most intriguing characteristics, and has triggered scientific research aiming to demonstrate specific molecular features that could explain mechanisms underneath the ability of tumor cells to detach from primary malignancy and gain excess to the surrounding structures.[6]

Although development of GEP-NETs is still unclear, significant breakthrough has been made in elucidating molecular genetics of neuroendocrine tumors exhibiting a hereditary background. Those rare tumor types (5-10% of all GEP-NETs) are often caused by mutations in tumor suppressor genes MEN1, VHL, NF-1, TSC1, and TSC2 which in turn lead to development of NETs as a part of multiple endocrine neoplasia type 1, von Hippel Lindau disease, neurofibromatosis type 1 and tuberous sclerosis complex respectively.[7] Besides tumor suppression genes, studies have also demonstrated involvement of oncogenes, each of which may be associated with several different abnormalities that include point mutations, gene deletions, DNA methylation, chromosomal losses and chromosomal gains (Figure 1).[3,8,9]

Perhaps the best characterized is the genetic background of the MEN1 syndrome, which in addition to neuroendocrine tumors of duodenum and pancreas includes adenomas/ hyperplasia of other endocrine glands (parathyroid hyperplasia/hyperparathyroidism, pituitary adenomas and adrenal cortical adenomas). It involves mutations of the MEN-1 tumor suppressor gene. This chromosome 11q13 gene encodes protein menin which interacts with a number of proteins involved in the transcriptional regulation and genome stability, so it has been proposed to be a key player in regulating NET cell proliferation.[8]

The *MEN-1* gene, although conferring a high disease risk in MEN-1 patients where it represents a putative tumor suppressor gene accounts for less than 40 percent of sporadic GEP-NET cases.[10] Thus, the genes involved in neuroendocrine tumorigenesis and the cellular roles of their proteins on proliferation and/or apoptotic pathways remain largely unknown. Studies of comparative genomic hybridization and allelic loss analysis have detected a large number of genomic regions with loss or gain of genetic material, further elucidating genetic differences between GEP-NETs of various primary localizations, and proving the heterogeneity of the tumors.[11]

In general, foregut GEP-NETs often show loss of 11q, while tumors of midgut origin frequently show losses on chromosome 18q. The genetic abnormalities in hindgut NETs have not been well characterized, but it was noticed that larger tumors tend to express transforming growth factor-alpha (TGF-α) more frequently, while epidermal growth factor receptor (EGFR) was expressed in all lesions.[12]

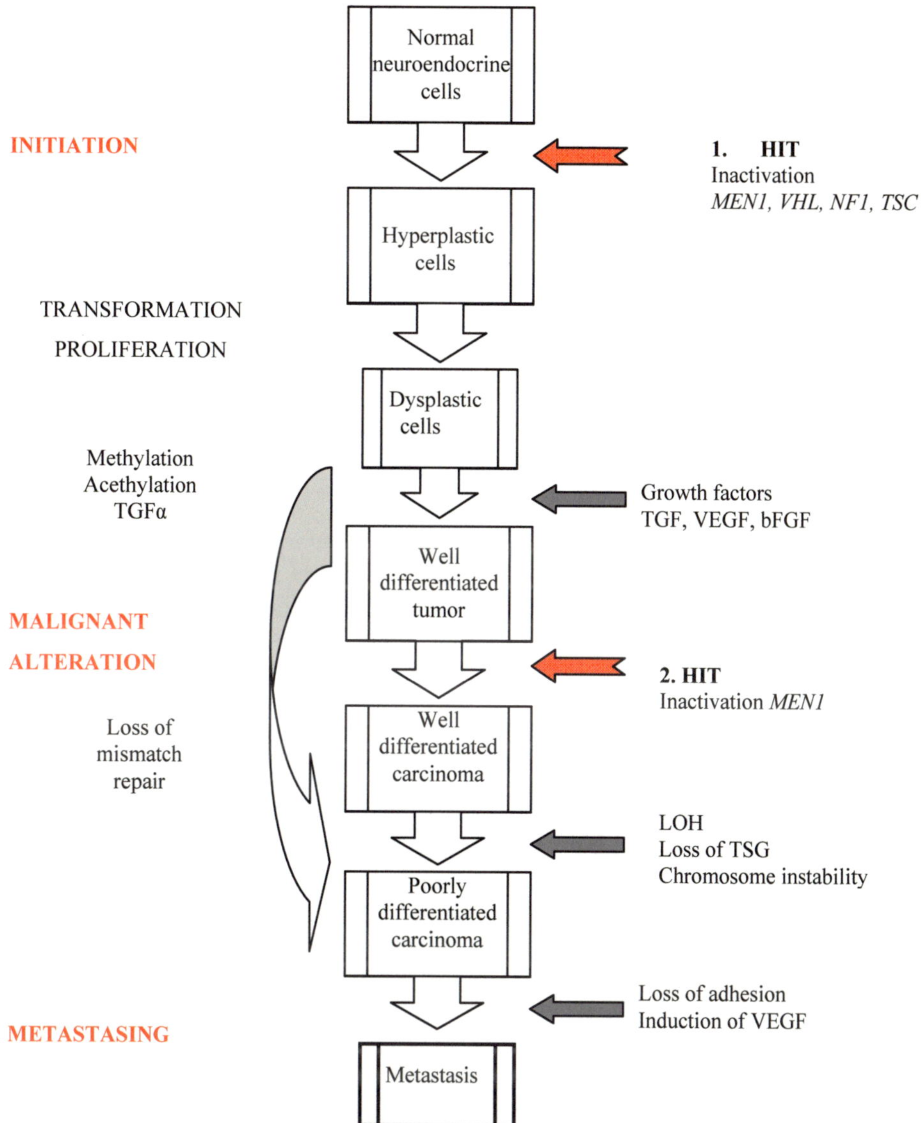

Fig. 1. Development of GEP-NETs.

Comparative studies of pancreatic adenocarcinoma and pancreatic neuroendocrine tumors (pNETs) have helped in giving insight into cellular biology of those specific tumors. Unlike pancreatic adenocarcinomas, pNETs do not exhibit mutations in K-Ras oncogene or p53 tumor suppressor gene, which are often mutated in the former. Also, the pattern of genomic alterations of pNETs differs from that of gastrointestinal NETs, where losses on chromosome 18q are almost a rule (occur in 38-88% of tumors).[13]

It seems that specifics of pNET development are gains and losses of chromosomes, which also appear to influence disease stage. Specifically, genomic gains are common on chromosomes 4pq, 5pq, 7pq, 9q, 12q, 14q, 17pq, 18q and 20q, while losses occur on chromosomes 1p, 3p, 6q, 10p, 11pq, X and Yq. It is interesting that nonfunctioning pNETs harbor more genetic changes than those functional; in particular they exhibit more losses of 3p and mutations in MEN1 gene. The locus 3p is especially interesting while it harbors several tumor suppressor genes like VHL and retinoic receptor-beta (RAR-β). The later, involved in induction of apoptosis, has been found hypermethylated in 25% of pNETS.[14]

In addition to tumor suppressor genes, some oncogenes have also been found altered in pNETs. Those specifically include over expression of growth factor-related genes such as insulin like growth factor binding protein 3 (IGFBP3), cell adhesion and migration molecules as well as endothelial elements, suggesting an important role of tumor microenvironment.[15]

Dysregulation of DNA methylation patterns is a central feature of colon carcinogenesis, and was also found to be present in development of gastrointestinal neuroendocrine tumors (especially carcinoids). This finding is interesting from the nutrigenomic point of view, and it raises the possibility of tumor prevention with folate and vitamin B12 supplementation.[16,17]

Positive immunohistochemistry staining for different cytokines and growth factors in the GEP-NETs as well as occurrence of GEP-NETs in the setting of inflammatory bowel disease led to the belief that chronic inflammation may play a crucial role in their development and that a number of more prevalent, low penetrance genes contribute to GEP-NET susceptibility in a larger population of patients.[18]

With respect to the role of inflammatory signals in promoting the development of cancer, there is now emerging evidence for an important relationship between macrophage migration inhibitory (MIF) factor expression, oncogenesis and tumor progression. It seems that in different tumors MIF directly promotes tumorigenesis by inhibiting p53 accumulation, promotes cellular proliferation through activation of members of the MAPK family and through induction of COX-2/PGE-2 influences tumor growth and viability. MIF was found to be co-secreted with adrenocorticotrophic hormone (ACTH) by the anterior pituitary, and it has the ability to override its antiinflammatory effects, thus promoting the inflammation and favouring protumor microinvironment.[19]

It seems that immune system through the network of different cytokines and growth factors may also play permissive role in GEP-NET development (Figure 2).[20]

It is now widely acknowledged that chronic inflammatory conditions can both pave the way for and sustain conditions favorable for carcinogenesis and tumor progression. Although the molecular mechanisms of this causal relationship remain to be elucidated, there is strong evidence of association between chronic inflammation and aproximately 1/5 of human cancers confirmed by numerous epidemiologic, gene association and molecular studies.[21]

Overall, it appears that chronic inflammation more often stimulates then inhibits tumor development. The persistence of chronic inflammation plays a critical role in initiating, sustaining and advancing tumor growth, and thus modulating the immune response may still be an alluring goal for therapeutic intervention.[22,23]

Although a pathogenic role for chronic inflammation has been suggested in multiple tumor systems in tumor initiation, progression and metastatic potential, the mechanism of this important association is still not understood completely. The development of a tumor is associated with the growth and expansion of not only tumor cells but also stroma, vessels and infiltrating inflammatory cells, and it is the interaction between these different cell types that propagates tumor growth. Cytokines found in tumors, acting on paracrine and autocrine loops, are most likely the key players in the mentioned communication[24], and for some of them link has been found between the serum and/or tumor tissue level and cancer survival.[25]

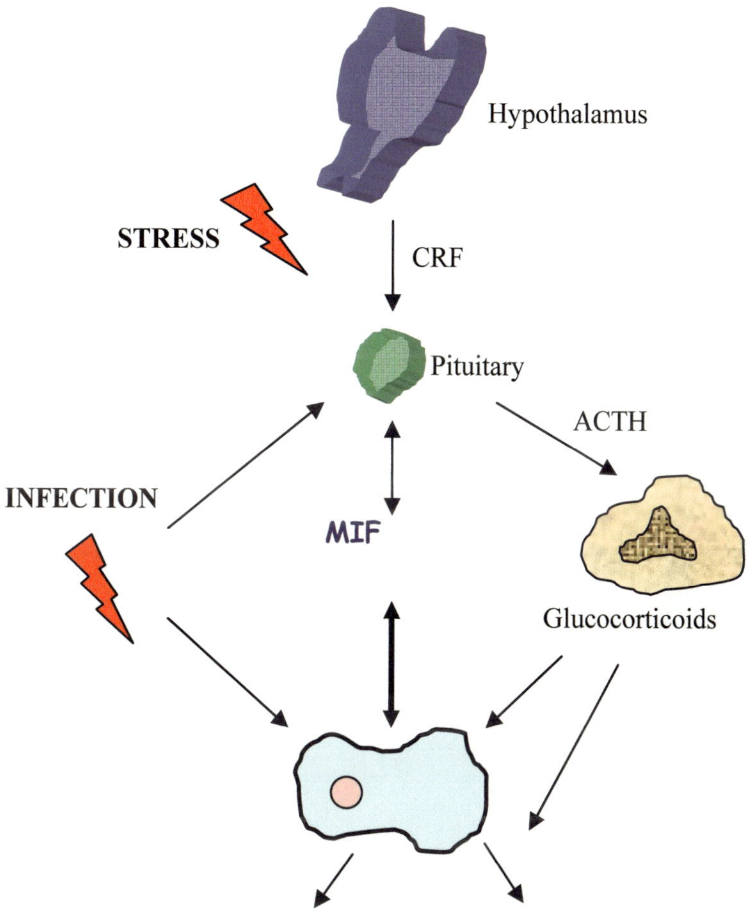

Fig. 2. Connection between the endocrine system and cytokines.

Cytokines and growth factors seem to largely contribute to the development and progression of GEP-NETs[13,17,26,27], but their involvement in the autocrine stimulation of tumor cells, either in genesis and/or in the progression of GEP-NETs has not yet been clearly elucidated.[28]

GEP-NETs represent a tumor entity with an extraordinary high vascularization along with an abundant production and secretion of growth factors, especially vascular endothelial growth factor (VEGF), epidermal growth factor (EGF), platelet-derived growth factor (PDGF), insulin like growth factor (IGF), fibroblast growth factor (FGF) and transforming growth factor-α (TGF-α), which according to both observational and mechanistic data connect chronic inflammation with gastrointestinal carcinogenesis.[20,23]

MEN-1 patients have a higher serum level of fibroblast growth factor (FGF), which correlates with the amount of tumor-associated fibroblastic response. Furthermore, insulin-like growth factor-I (IGF-I) receptors found on GEP-NET cells suggest an autocrine trophic function for the mentioned growth factor in these tumors.[27] Patients with carcinoid syndrome were found to have positive immunohistochemistry for TGF -β on the right sided heart valves, as a consequence of NET progression and metastasis.[29]

For further cancer evolution angiogenesis plays an important role. Proinflammatory cytokines such as tumor necrosis factor-α (TNF-α), IL1 and IL6 once again participate in this process by inducing the production of angiogenic factors, mainly VEGF. The role of vascular endothelial growth factor (VEGF) in the new vessel formation of these highly vascularized tumors is increasingly studied, and it appears to be involved in the metastasing process of the mentioned tumors. Higher levels of cytokines and growth factors detected in GEP-NETs are responsible for neurotrophic effects, smooth muscle cell hypertrophy and proliferation of both intimal and adventitial elastic tissue of the mesenteric blood vessels leading to vascular elastosis sometimes associated with ischemic changes of the near-by tissue (Figure 3).[6,30]

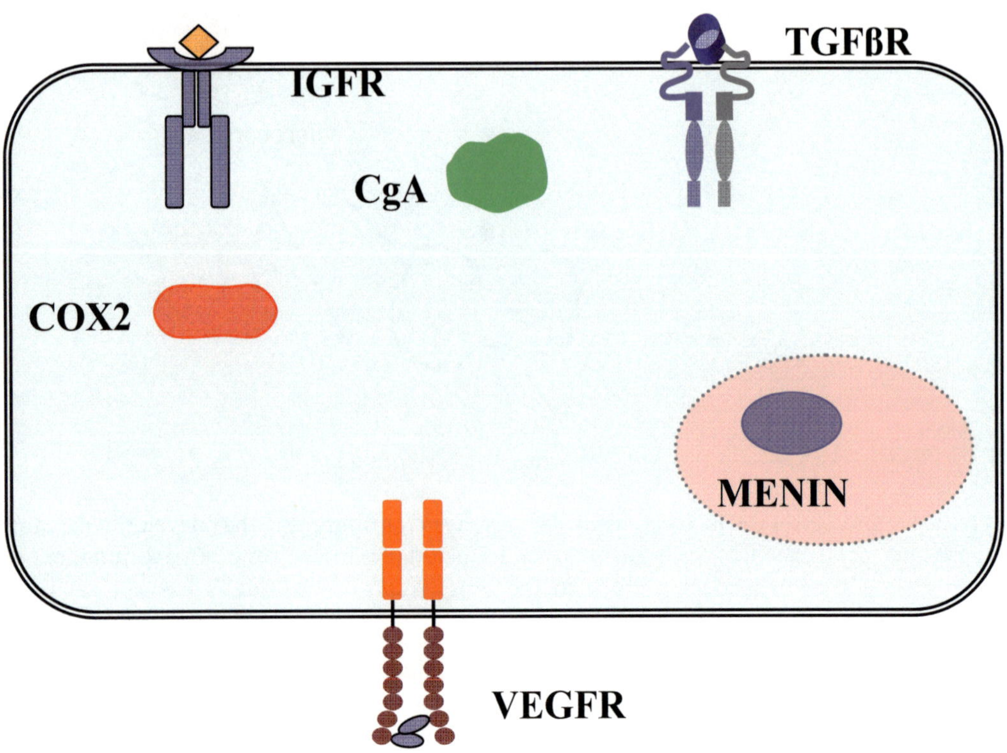

Fig. 3. Tumor cell markers of neuroendocrine cell.

Cytokine genes are highly polymorphic, with polymorphisms frequently located in regions of DNA that regulate transcription, or posttranscriptional events, thus influencing functional activity. Recently published studies connected proinflammatory cytokine genes SNPs with cancer susceptibility and severity, putting them in the spot light as cancer-modifier genes.[31] This is particularly true for cytokine gene polymorphisms and gastrointestinal malignancy, where many authors suggest the role of inflammation-mediated oncogenesis.[16,18,32] It seems likely that they also contribute to GEP-NET development.[33,34]

Genetic polymorphisms directly influence interindividual variation in the cytokine response, and this clearly contributes to an individual's ultimate clinical outcome. Many single nucleotide polymorphisms (SNPs) have been detected within the cytokine gene sequences, particularly within the promoter regions. Several of these SNPs may be associated with differential level of gene transcription, thus influencing levels of cytokines and growth factors in sera and tumor tissue and ultimately altering the disease prognosis by influencing anti-tumor immunologic response or pathways of (neo)angiogenesis.

However, for the ultimate outcome, not only cytokines or growth factors but also (tumor) cell type and stimulus may also be important.[35] In our investigation of the role of IL-6 in GEP-NETs we have found the significantly higher proportion of high expression genotypes (*-174 C/G* and *G/G*) in the nonfunctioning pNETs, discriminating them from functional pNETs and gastrointestinal NETs (mainly of midgut origin). Mentioned patients had also higher concentrations of IL-6 in their sera (it was overall elevated in 36.8% of patients), suggesting the potential role of IL-6 as a novel diagnostic and prognostic marker of nonfunctioning pNETs.[36]

A number of studies have reported associations between TNF-α promoter SNPs with high expression alleles (*-238A, -308A, -1031C*) and susceptibility to cancer.[20,37] Our ongoing studies have strongly confirmed the role of TNF-α *-1031C* (high expression) allele as a potential risk factor for developing GEP-NET. Also, we have found the higher level of the *-308* high expression genotypes (*AG, AA*) as well as high expression *-308A* allele among the patients contracting foregut GEP-NETs than in those with midgut tumors. This finding may provide better insight in the role of cytokines in the development of different GEP-NET types and differentiation, and possibly open new prospective in GEP-NET treatment.[38]

2. References

[1] Plöckinger U, Rindi G, Arnold A, Eriksson B, Krenning EP, DeHerder WW, Goede A, Caplin Guidelines for the Diagnosis and Treatment of Neuroendocrine Gastrointestinal Tumors. Neuroendocrinology 2004;80:394-424.

[2] Cigrovski Berković M, Altabas V, Herman D, Hrabar D, Goldoni V, Vizner B, Zjačić-Rotkvić V. A Single-Centre Experience with Octreotide in the Treatment of Different Hypersecretory Syndromes in Patients with Functional Gastroenteropancreatic Neuroendocrine Tumors. Coll Antropol. 2007;31:531-534.

[3] Rindi G, Bordi C. Highlights of the biology of endocrine tumors of the gut and pancreas. Endocrine-Related Cancer 2003;10:427-436.

[4] Ardill JE. Circulating markers for endocrine tumors of the gastroenteropancreatic tract. Ann Clin Biochem 2008;45:539-559.

[5] Cigrovski Berkovic M, Jokic M, Zjacic-Rotkvic V, Kapitanovic S. The role of cytokines and their polymorphisms in the gastroenteropancreatic neuroendocrine tumors (GEP-NETs): mini review. Periodicum Biologorum. 2007;109:111-114.

[6] Delle Fave G, Corleto VD. Oncogenes, growth factors, receptor expression and proliferation markers in digestive neuroendocrine tumors. A critical reappraisal. Ann of Oncol 2001;12 (suppl 2):S13-S17.

[7] Zikusoka MN, Kidd M, Eick G, Latich I, Modlin IM. The molecular genetics of gastroenteropancreatic neuroendocrine tumors. Cancer 2005;04:2292-2309.

[8] Perren A, Komminoth P, Heitz PU. Molecular genetics of gastroenteropancreatic endocrine tumors. Ann NY Acad Sci 2004;1014:199-208.

[9] Chan AO, Kim SG, Bedeir A, Issa JP, Hamilton SR, Rashid A 2003 CpG island methylation in carcinoid and pancreatic endocrine tumors. Oncogene 22:924-934.

[10] Pannett AA, Thakker RV 2001 Somatic mutations in MEN type 1 tumors, consistent with the Knudson "two-hit" hypothesis. J Clin Endocrinol Metab 86:4371-4374.

[11] Duerr E-M, Chung DC. Molecular Genetics of pancreatic neuroendocrine tumors. In: A century of advances in neuroendocrine tumor biology and treatment. (Ed. Modlin IM, Oberg K.), Felsenstein C.C.C.P. 2007.

[12] Leotlela PD, Jauch A, Holtgrave-Grez H, Thakker RV. Genetics of neuroendocrine tumors and carcinoid tumors. Endocrine Related Cancer 2003;10:437-450.

[13] Öberg K. Carcinoid tumors-current considerations. In: A century of advances in neuroendocrine tumor biology and treatment. (Ed. Modlin IM, Oberg K.), Felsenstein C.C.C.P. 2007.

[14] Speel EJ et al. Genetic evidence for early divergence of small functioning and nonfunctioning endocrine pancreatic tumors: gain of 9Q34 is an early event in insulinomas. Cancer Res 2001;61(13):5186-92.

[15] Östman A. Tumor stroma-a perspective of therapeutic and prognostic opportunities. In: A century of advances in neuroendocrine tumor biology and treatment. (Ed. Modlin IM, Oberg K.), Felsenstein C.C.C.P. 2007.

[16] House MG et al. Aberrant hypermethylation of tumor suppresor genes in pancreatic endocrine neoplasms. Ann Surg 2003;238(3):423-31.

[17] Shimizu T et al. Growth characteristics of rectal carcinoid tumors. Oncology 2000;59:229-237.

[18] Terris B et al. Expression of vascular endothelial growth factor in digestive neuroendocrine tumors. Histopathology 1998; 32:133-138.

[19] Conroy H, Mawhinney L, S. C. Donnelly SC. Inflammation and cancer: macrophage migration inhibitory factor (MIF)—the potential missing link. Q J Med 2010; 103:831–836.

[20] Wulbrand U, Wied M, Zofel P, Goke B, Arnold R, Fehmann HC. Growth factor receptor expression in human gastroenteropancreatic neuroendocrine tumors. European J of Clin Invest 1998;28:1038-1049.

[21] De Marzo AM et al. Inflammation in prostate carcinogenesis. Nat Rev Cancer 2007;7:256–269.

[22] Jackson L, Evers BM. Chronic inflammation and pathogenesis of GI and pancreatic cancers. Cancer Treat Res 2006;130:39-65.

[23] Höpfner M, Schuppan D, Scherübl H. Treatment of gastrointestinal neuroendocrine tumors with inhibitors of growth factor receptors and their signaling pathways: Recent advances and future perspectives. World J Gastroenterol 2008;14(16):2461-2473.

[24] Gonda TA, Tu S, Wang TC. Chronic inflammation, the tumor microenvironment and carcinogenesis. Cell cycle 2009;8 (13):2005-13.

[25] Westbrook AM, Szakmary A, Schiestl RH. Mechanisms of intestinal inflammation and development of associated cancers: Lessons learned from mouse models. Mutat Res 2010;705(1):40-59.

[26] Wiedenmann B, Pape UF 2004 From basic to clinical research in gastroenteropancreatic neuroendocrine tumor disease-the clinician-scientist perspective. Neuroendocrinology 80(suppl 1):94-98.

[27] Wild A et al. Frequent methylation-associated silencing of the tissue inhibitor of metalloproteinase-3 gene in pancreatic endocrine tumors. J Clin Endocrinol Metab 2003; 88:1367-1373.

[28] Barakat MT, Meeren K, Bloom SR. Neuroendocrine tumors. Endocrine-Related Cancer 2004;11:1-18.

[29] Lester WM, Gotlieb AI 1991 The cardiovascular system. In *Functional Endocrine Pathology*, vol. 2, pp 724-747. Eds k Kovacs and SL Asa, Boston: Blackwell

[30] Ardill JES, Erikkson B. The importance of the measurment of circulating markers in patients with neuroendocrine tumors of the pancreas and gut. Endocrine-related Cancer 2003;10:459-462.

[31] Seike M et al. Use of a cytokine gene expression signature in lung adenocarcinoma and the surrounding tissue as a prognostic classifier. J Natl Cancer Inst 2007;99:1257-1269.

[32] Bidwell J et al. Cytokine gene polymorphism in human disease: on-line databases. Genes Immun 1999;1:3-19.

[33] Wilkening S et al. Interleukin promoter polymorphisms and prognosis in colorectal cancer. Carcinogenesis 2008;29(6):1202-1206.

[34] Cigrovski Berkovic M. The role of cytokines and growth factors in development and progression of gastroenteropancreatic neuroendocrine tumors (GEP-NETs). Doctoral thesis. University of Zagreb, 2009.

[35] MacArthur M, Hold GL, El-Omar EM. Inflammation and Cancer II. Role of chronic inflammation and cytokine gene polymorphisms in the pathogenesis of gastrointestinal malignancy. Am J Physiol Gastrointest Liver Physiol 2004;286:G515-G520.

[36] Cigrovski Berković M, Jokić M, Marout J, Radošević S, Zjačić-Rotkvić V, Kapitanović, S. IL-6-174 C/G polymorphism in the gastroenteropancreatic neuroendocrine tumors (GEP-NETs). Experimental and Molecular Pathology 2007;83:474-479.

[37] Anderson GM, Nakada MT, Dewitte M. Tumor necrosis factor-α in the pathogenesis and treatment of cancer. Curr Opin Pharmacol 2004; 4314-4320.

[38] Berkovic M, Cacev T, Zjacic-Rotkvic V, Kapitanovic S. TNF-α promoter SNPs in gastroenteropancreatic neuroendocrine tumors (GEP-NET). Neuroendocrinology 2006;84:346-352.

2

Chromogranin A and Neuroendocrine Tumors

Angela Prestifilippo, Giusi Blanco,
Maria Paola Vitale and Dario Giuffrida
Istituto Oncologico del Mediterraneo, Viagrande - CT
Italy

1. Introduction

Neuroendocrine tumors (NETs) are neoplasms that arise from cells of the endocrine and nervous systems. Many are benign, while some are cancers. They most commonly occur in the intestine, but are also found in the lung and in the rest of the body.

A neuroendocrine tumor is suspected when classical clinical symptoms occur but the large majority of NETs does not show any specific symptomatology (Oberg et al., 1999). Accordingly, the biochemical diagnosis is of great value, with the validation of radio-immunoenzymatic assays for various circulating peptide hormones in the last decade, clinical awareness and ability to diagnose NET is increased . However, due to the relative low incidence of NETs and the very large number of measurable hormones, clinicians need to know which measurable variables have an established clinical value and are cost effective (Giuffrida et al., 2006)

Neuroendocrine tumors can be functional and nonfunctional.

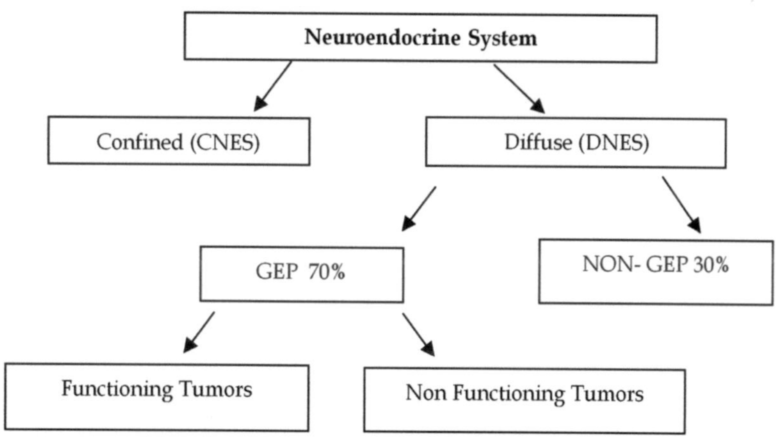

Fig. 1. Neuroendocrine System GEP: Gastroenteropancreatic

In the case of funtional NETs signs and symptoms include:

- Flushing of the face and neck (appearance of deep red color, usually with sudden onset)
- Diarrhea, nausea, vomiting, rapid heart rate

- Wheezing, coughing, difficulty breathing

2. Tumor markers

Symptoms that are exhibited in the functional NETs is related to the release of circulating hormones and peptides such as catecholamines, insulin, 5-hydroxyindoleacetic acid (5-HIAA), gastrin, calcitonin and others. Although there are many kinds of NETs, they are treated as a group because the cells of these neoplasms share common features, such as looking similar, having special secretory granules, and often producing biogenic amines and polypeptide hormones 5-hydroxytryptamine (5-HT) or serotonin is product by functional neuroendocrine tumors (NETs) originating from the midgut. Serotonin is a tryptophan-derived biogenic amine involved in smooth muscle contraction, blood pressure regulation and both peripheral and central nervous system neurotransmission. Approximately 2% of dietary tryptophan is converted into serotonin. Serotonin is synthesized and stored in enterochromaffin cells of the gastrointestinal tract (80% of total body serotonin content), in dense granules of platelets (storage only) and in the serotoninergic neurons of the central nervous system. The urinary breakdown metabolite of serotonin is 5-hydroxyindole acetic acid (5 - HIAA) which is particularly useful in the diagnosis and follow-up of NETs with carcinoid syndrome. Serum measurements of serotonin are possible in these patients; however, large individual variation makes them unreliable for diagnosis and in follow-up. Universally, 5-HIAA is the most frequently performed assay in the clinical setting of the carcinoid syndrome (O'Toole et al., 2009).

The generic markers of NETs are Neurone Specific Enolase (NSE) and Cromogranine A. Neurone-Specific Enolase is an useful immunohistochemical marker of NETs. Neverthelles ,its serum mesurament has not, except for patients with small cell lung cancer and neuroblastoma, because of relatively low sensitivity and specificity of the marker (Giovannella et al., 1999).

3. Chromogranin

Chromogranin A is an acidic glycoprotein expressed in the secretory granules of most normal and neoplastic neuroendocrine cell types, where it is released togheter with peptide hormones and biogenic amines. In humans, chromogranin A protein is encoded by the CHGA gene (Helman et al., 1988)

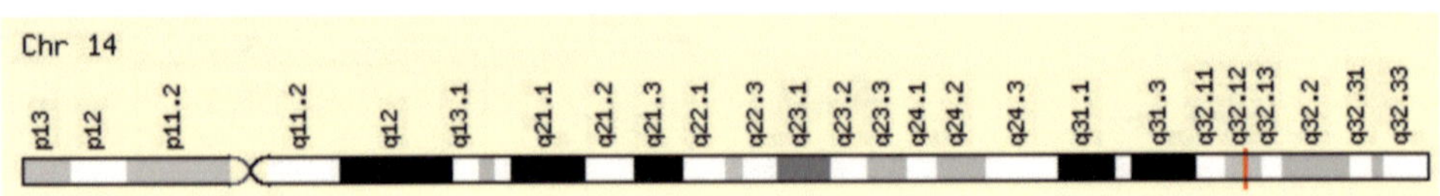

Fig. 2. CHGA structure

The chromogranin family consists of at least three different watersoluble acidic glycoproteins (CgA, CgB, and secretogranin II, sometimes called chromogranin C). Upon stimulation, CgA and other peptide hormones and neuropeptides are released. CgA is also secreted from neuroendocrine derived tumors including foregut, midgut and hindgut gastrointestinal NETs, pheochromocytomas, neuroblastomas, medullary thyroid carcinomas, some pituitary tumors, functioning and non-functioning pancreatic NETs and other amine precursor uptake and decarboxylation tumors.

Chromogranin A might promote the generation of secretory granules. Chromogranin A is the precursor to several functional peptides including vasostatin, pancreastatin, catestatin and parastatin. These peptides negatively modulate the neuroendocrine function of the releasing cell (autocrine) or nearby cells (paracrine). Other peptides derived from chromogranin A with uncertain function include chromostatin, WE-14 and GE-25.

Chromogranin A concentrations are normally low. An increased level in a symptomatic person may indicate the presence of a tumor but not what type it is or where it is. The quantity of CgA is not associated with the severity of the symptoms but with the mass and the functional activity of the tumor (Wu et al., 2000)

The possibility to measure Chromogranin A (CgA) plasma levels by means of radio- or immunoenzymatic assay represents a tremendous step forward in the management of patients with NETs.

3.1 Chromogranin: Laboratory test

Chromogranin can be dosed. The IRMA method is based on two monoclonal antibodies raised against the unprocessed central domain of the human CgA, allowing sensitive detection of total human CgA. Recombinant human CgA was used as calibrator and the standard curve concentration ranged from 22 to 1200 ng/ml, with a minimal detectable level of 10ng/ml. Inter-assay coefficients of variation were 3.4 and 4.5% at 124.7and 355.2 ng/ml, respectively. Intra-assay coefficients of variation were 5.1, 3.0, and 7.8% for the following ranges 15-25, 90-110, and 500-700ng/ml, respectively.

The ELISA assay is based on two polyclonal rabbit antibodies directed toward a 23 kDa carboxyl-terminal fragment of human CgA, therefore measuring more human CgA fragments . The calibrators were extracted from urine of patients with carcinoids and the standard curve concentraction ranged from 5 to 650 U/l, with a minimal detectable level of 5U/l. Inter-assay coefficients of variation were 3.4, 3.9 and 6.8 at 11.5, 52.7, and 358U/l, respectively. Intra-assay coefficients of variation were 4.5, 3.8 and 8.5% for the following ranges 5-10, 15-25 and 250-450 U/l, respectively (Zatelli et al., 2007). The three most commonly available employed assays for CgA measurement, has been compared in a group of NET patients and has been found that sensitivities vary between 67 and 93%, while specificities were 1 to 85% for all three (Stridsberg et al., 2003). A recent multicenter prospective comparison between two methods, immunoradiometric and ELISA, found a 36% clinical discordance rate. These results were mirrored with a difference of 5-fold inter-laboratory variation rate in a recent Italian study aimed at assessing CgA detection performance as applied to immunoradiometric and ELISA assays (Janson et al., 1997). A further prospective analysis underlined CgA to be a practical marker in patients with NET, however, with limited diagnostic power. A cut-off of 53 ng/ml for IRMA and 16 U/l for ELISA for discriminating between healthy controls and NET patients yielded only moderate sensitivities (71.3 and 83%, respectively) and specificities (71 and 85%, respectively).

3.2 Chromogranin related to net

The Chromogranin A test is used often as a tumor marker. It may be ordered in combination with or in place of 5-HIAA to help diagnose carcinoid tumors. It is also used to help monitor the effectiveness of treatment and detect recurrence of this tumor. Sometimes it may be ordered with specific hormones, such as catecholamines, to help diagnose and monitor a pheochromocytoma. It may also be used to detect the presence of other neuroendocrine tumors, even those that do not secrete hormones . Plasma CgA levels (2-18 u/l) were found elevated in a variety of NETs, including pheocromocytoma, carcinoid tumors, pancreatic islet cell tumors, medullary carcinoma of the thyroid, small-cell lung cancer and so forth (Verderio et al., 2007).

Positive Cromogranin A related to Neuroendocrine Tumors:

- Gastroenteropancreatic NETs
- Anterior Pituitary tumors
- Parathyroid tumors
- Medullary Thyroid Carcinoma
- Merkel Cell Tumor
- Ectopic Adrenocorticotropic Hormone Producing Tumors
- Ganglioneuroma / Neuroblastoma
- Pheocromocytoma
- Small Cell Lung Cancer
- Prostate Cancer

Table 1. CgA and Neuroendocrine Tumors

The sensitivity and specificity of circulating CgA in any NETs vary between 70% and 95%. The highest accuracy has been observed in tumors characterized by an intense secretory activity, but its specificity and sensitivity remain very high also in non-functioning tumors.

Although CgA specificity cannot compete with that of the specific hormonal products secreted by many NETs, this molecule has very useful clinical applications in subjects with NETs for whom either no marker is available or the marker is inconvenient for routine clinical use generally, if concentrations of CgA are elevated prior the treatment and then fall, the treatment is likely to have been effective. CgA concentrations may be elevated but not monitored with conditions, such as liver disease, inflammatory bowel disease, renal insufficiency, and with stress. These possible causes for elevated CgA levels should be considered when interpreting test results, as false positive.

Overall CgA has been found to be clinically informative and moderately sensitive in the majority of studies devoted to this topic. CgA was found of a large mixed NET patient cohort, CgA was more sensitive than neurone-specific enolase (Baudin et al., 1998) . While performances have been limited in low-level cut-offs due to the overlap with control populations, very high levels of serum CgA are rarely found outside the setting of NETs with the exception of patients on gastric acid secretory blockers, especially PPIs (Sanduleanu et al., 2001) or those with hypergastrinaemia. Specificity of CgA in the diagnosis of NETs depends on the tumor type and burden (100% specificities have been reported in patients with metastatic disease), the quality of the control populations used and the cut-off values employed. Elevated CgA was found to be more sensitive than high urinary 5- HIAA levels in patients with metastatic midgut lesions (87 vs. 76%, respectively). A significant positive relation between the serum levels of CgA and the tumor mass in NETs, has been demonstrated; however, the distinction between high and low tumor volume may be open to question, infact, high CgA concentrations were found in all patients with gastrinoma, although tumor was small in volume (Nobels et al., 1997). In a mixed series of 128 patients with NET, increased CgA levels were found in 29% and 67% of patients with locoregional or metastatic disease, respectively. Nonetheless, the prognostic value of CgA in patients with NET has not been confirmed to date.

False-positive elevation of CgA may occur in the following circumstances:

- Impaired renal function
- Parkinson disease
- Untreated hypertension
- Pregnancy
- Chronic atrophic gastritis (type A)
- Treatment with anti-secretory medications, expecially PPIs

Chronic elevation of gastrin levels provokes hyperplasia of the neuroendocrine cells of the stomach, and these cells are able to secrete CgA (D'Adda et al., 1990) . In patients with chronically elevated CgA and Zollinger Ellison Syndrome (ZES), has been demonstrated that the CgA concentrations can be normalized by gastrectomy alone, without resection of the gastrin producing tumor. A more recently described case report of false-positive CgA was due to the presence of heterophile antibodies (HAb), which can bind to animal antigens and may be present in up to 40% of the normal population (Levinson et al., 2007); in the CgA immunometric assays, HAb interferences may be circumnavigated by using a Habblocking tube.

CgA laboratory tests that have been developed and validated will all be slightly different, and their results will not be interchangeable. For this reason, if someone is having more than one CgA test performed (such as for monitoring), all test are sent to the same laboratory.

The very frequent elevation of CgA in patients with pheochromocytomas/paragangliomas confirms that it may be the marker of choice for these diseases, being more convenient than catecholamines either measured in plasma or in urine.

The highest CgA levels were noted in patients with metastatic carcinoid tumors and neuroendocrine carcinomas of gastrointestinal origin. Conversely, the lowest values were found in patients with advanced SCLC. Some data support the notion that CgA is less useful in undifferentiated neuroendocrine neoplasms (Blanco, 2007; Stivanello, 2011).

It is noteworthy that elevated plasma CgA levels cannot differentiate between neuroendocrine and non neuroendocrine neoplasms. Slightly elevated CgA levels, in fact, were identified in more than 40% of patients with advanced non-endocrine tumors, a proportion that was not so different from that of patients with SCLC (Nobels, 1997, Stivanello, 2001). The detection of elevated plasma CgA in non-endocrine tumors mainly indicates that there is a neuroendocrine differentiation and a proliferation of neuroendocrine cells at advanced stage of many carcinomas.

Drugs that stimulate secretion of neuroendocrine cells can lead to artifactual chromogranin A elevations. In particular, proton pump inhibitors (e.g., omeprazole), which are used in the treatment of esophageal and gastroduodenal ulcer disease and dyspepsia, will result in significant elevations of serum chromogranin A levels, often to many times above the normal range. If medically feasible, proton pump inhibitor therapy should be discontinued drug week of serum chromogranin A levels.

Chromogranin A and its peptide fragments are cleared by a combination of hepatic metabolism and renal excretion. In patients with significant impairment of liver or kidney function, serum chromogranin levels are often substantially elevated and single chromogranin A measurements are uninterpretable. Serial measurements may have some value in selected patients if the disturbance in hepatic or renal function remains stable, but results must be interpreted with extreme caution. There is no universal calibration standard for serum chromogranin A assays. In addition, different chromogranin A assays, which use different antibodies or antibody combinations, will display different cross-reactivity with the various chromogranin A fragments. Therefore, reference intervals and individual patient results differ significantly between different chromogranin A assays and cannot be directly compared. Serial measurements should be performed with the same assay, or, if assays are changed, patients should be rebaselined. As with all immunometric assays, there is a low but definite possibility of false-positive results in patients with heterophile antibodies.

These antibodies are rarely found in the normal population, but are observed at increased rates in persons with autoimmune disease or after prior sensitization to rodent proteins (patients who have received diagnostic or therapeutic mouse monoclonal antibodies). Blocking reagents have been added to this assay to minimize the likelihood of heterophile antibody interference. However, test results that do not fit the clinical picture should always be discussed with the laboratory.

A "hook effect" can occur at extremely high chromogranin A concentrations, resulting in a lower measured chromogranin A concentration than is actually contained in the specimen. This is not expected to impact the utility of the assay for initial diagnosis, as levels will typically remain significantly above the reference range, even in the presence of hooking. However, hooking may complicate the interpretation of serial chromogranin A measurements in rare patients with extremely high levels. Normally it would be useful to dose dilute and remeasure all specimens >625 ng/mL to minimize the risk of this occurring. However, if there is the clinical suspicion of hooking, then retesting after further specimen dilution should be requested.

There are some pitfalls in the interpretation of CgA levels. Among them, renal impairment is one of the most important. All the patients with chronic renal failure presented very high levels of CgA, thus suggesting that serum creatinine should always be measured concomitantly with plasma CgA (Stridsberg et al., 2003)

Circulating CgA was found to be a reliable marker for the follow-up of patients with neuroendocrine tumors. CgA levels were with not evident disease (NED) , CgA levels were within normality. In advanced cases submitted to systemic treatment, a clear relationship was found between changes in CgA levels and disease response. This marker decreased in all patients showing a tumour shrinkage after cytotoxic treatment, increased in the great majority of patients showing progressive disease, and did not change in most cases depicting a disease stabilization. Discrepancies between tumor and biochemical changes in non-responding patients are attributable to the concomitant administration of somatostatin analog (Campana et al., 2007)

The correlation between CgA levels and tumor mass is lost during treatment with somatostatin so that CgA may not be used as a marker of tumor response when a cytotoxic regimen is administered in combination with a somatostatin analog (O'Toole et al., 2009).

4. Conclusion

Many data confirm the general view that CgA is the best circulating neuroendocrine marker available up to now. Its clinical application involves all differentiated NETs, irrespective of tumor location and functional status. In gastrointestinal neuroendocrine tumours the measurement of general and specific markers offers important information for the clinician treating patients. This information is useful for the initial diagnosis and during the follow-up for monitoring patients with non functional disease and under medical treatment. Several of the markers are good prognostic markers for both carcinoid and pancreatic disease (Ardill & Erikkson , 2003).

This marker seems to be less useful in undifferentiated tumors such as Small Cell Lung Cancer. Elevated CgA plasma levels allow the identification of the coexistence of neuroendocrine differentiation in the context of non-endocrine malignancies and this could have diagnostic, prognostic, and possibly therapeutic implications. A dynamic evaluation of this marker in the follow-up of NETs provides useful information on the disease recurrence in NED cases or on the treatment efficacy in advanced cases submitted to cytotoxic or biologic therapy (Zatelli et al., 2007)

CgA: General Remarks and Assays

- Elevated CgA can occur in normal individuals and in patients with non-NET tumors although the levels are usually lower than in patients with NET
- CgA is the most practical and useful general serum tumor marker in patients with NET
- Sensitivity of elevated CgA varies according to NET tumor type and volume
- Reference laboratories should be preferred for clinical samples assays
- Reference intervals and individual patient results differ significantly between different chromogranin A assays and cannot be directly compared
- Serial measurements should be performed using the same assay
- If assays are changed, patients should undergo a new baseline measurement
- False-positive results are possible in patients with hypergastrinaemia (especially on anti- secretory medications or chronic atrophic gastritis type A) and in the presence of heterophile antibodies (care in patients autoimmune disease or those sensitized to rodent proteins (mouse monoclonal antibodies))
- Where possible, proton pump inhibitors should be interrupted, leaving a clearance of at least 3 half-lives, prior to CgA plasma sampling.

5. References

Ardill, J.E.S. & Erikkson,B (2003). The importance of the measurement of circulating markers in patients with neuroendocrine tumours of the pancreas and gut, *Endocrine-Related Cancer,* Vol. 10, pp.459-642

Arnaldi, G., Cardinaletti, M. & Polenta, B. (2007). Biological markers of neuroendocrine tumors: false positives and negatives , Rivista Medica, Vol .13, No.2, pp.15-21

Baudin, E., Gigliotti, A. & Ducreux, M. (1998). Neuron-specific enolase and chromogranin A asmarkers of neuroendocrine tumours, *British Journal of cancer,* Vol .78, pp.1102–1107

Blanco,G., Martino, M., & Giuffrida, D. (2007). Clinical and therapeutical approach in poorly differentiated neuroendocrine tumors, *Rivista Medica,* Vol.13, No. 2,pp. 51-54

Campana, D., Nori, F. ,& Tomassetti, P. (2007). Chromogranin A: Is It a Useful Marker of Neuroendocrine Tumors, *Journal of Clinical Oncology,* Vol.25, No. 15, pp.1967-1973

D'Adda, T. Corleto,V. & Pilato, FP. (1990). Quantitative ultrastructure of endocrine cells of oxyntic mucosa in Zollinger-Ellison syndrome. Correspondence with light microscopic findings, *Gastroenterology,* Vol.99, pp. 17–26

Giovanella, L., La Rosa, S. & Garancini, S.(1999). Chromogranin-A as a serum marker for neuroendocrine tumors: comparison with neuron-specific enolase and correlation with immunohistochemical findings, *The international Journal of Biological Markers*, Vol.14, pp. 160–166

Giuffrida, D., Blanco,G. & Mare, M. (2006).A Clinical Approach to Neuroendocrine Tumors, *Supportive and Palliative Cancer Care*, Vol.2, No. 2, pp.17-19

Helman, LJ., Ahn, TG. & Israel, MA. (1988). Molecular cloning and primary structure of human chromogranin A (secretory protein I) cDNA, *Journal of Biological Chemistry* Vol.263, No. 23, pp. 11559–63

Hsiao, RJ., Mezger, MS. & O'Connor, DT. (1990). Chromogranin A in uremia: progressive retention of immunoreactive fragments, *Kidney International*, Vol.37, pp. 955–964

Janson, ET., Holmberg, L.& Stridsberg, M., (1997). Carcinoid tumors: analysis of prognostic factors and survival in 301 patients from a referral center, *Annals of Oncology*, Vol. 8, pp. 685–690

Levinson, SS. & Miller, JJ. (2002). Towards a better understanding of heterophile (and the like) antibody interference with modern immunoassays, *Clinica Chimica Acta Elsevier*, Vol. 325, pp. 1–15

Nobels, FR., Kwekkeboom, DJ. & Coopmans, W. (1997). Chromogranin A as serum marker for neuroendocrine neoplasia: comparison with neuron-specific enolase and the subunit of glycoprotein hormones, *Journal Clinical Endocrinology and metabolism*, Vol.82, pp. 2622–2628

Oberg, K., Janson, ET. & Eriksson ,B. (1999) Tumour markers in neuroendocrine tumours, *Italian Journal Gastroenterology and Hepatology*, Vol.31, pp.160-162 (suppl 2)

O' Toole, D., Grossman, A. & al other Mallorca Consensus Conference Partecipans (2009) ENETS Guidelines for the standards of care in neuroendocrine tumors biochemical markers, *Neuroendocrinology*, Vol. 90, pp. 194-202

Sanduleanu, S., De Bruïne,A .& Stockbrügger, RW.(2001). Serum chromogranin A as a screening test for gastric enterochromaffin-like cell hyperplasia during acid-suppressive therapy,*European Journal Clinical of Investigation*, Vol. 31, No.9, pp. 802-11

Stivanello, M., Berruti, A. & An & Dogliotti, L. (2001). Circulating chromogranin A in the assessment of patients with neuroendocrine tumours. A single institution experience, *Annals of Oncology* Vol. 12, supp l.2, pp.73-77

Stridsberg, M., Husebye, ES. (1997). Chromogranin A and chromogranin B are sensitive circulating markers for phaeochromocytoma, *European Journal of endocrinology*, Vol. 36, pp. 67–73

Stridsberg, M., Eriksson, B. & Janson, ET. (2003). A comparison between three commercial kits for chromogranin A measurements,*Journal Endocrinology*, Vol. 177, pp. 337–341

Verderio, P. Dittadi, R. & Marubini, E. (2007). An Italian program of external quality control for chromogranin A (CgA) assay: performance evaluation of CgA determination, *Clinical Chemistry and Laboratory Medicine* , Vol. 45, pp. 1244–1250

Wu, JT., Erickson, AJ. & Sun, CF. (2000). Elevated serum chromogranin A is detectable in patients with carcinomas at advanced disease stages, *Annals of Clinical and laboratory Science*, Vol. 30, No.2, pp. 175–8

Zatelli, M.C., Torta, M . & On behalf of the Italian CromoNet Working Group (2007). Chromogranin A as a marker of neuroendocrine neoplasia: an Italian Multicenter Study,*Endocrine-Related Cancer*, Vol. 14, pp.473.482

3

Circulating Markers in Gastroenteropancreatic Neuroendocrine Tumors (GEP NETs)

Sara Massironi[1], Matilde Pia Spampatti[1,2],
Roberta Elisa Rossi[1,2], Dario Conte[1,2], Clorinda Ciafardini[1,2],
Federica Cavalcoli[1] and Maddalena Peracchi[2]
[1]*Gastroenterology Unit II,*
Fondazione IRCCS Ca' Granda – Ospedale Maggiore Policlinico, Milano,
[2]*Postgraduate School of Gastroenterology, Università degli Studi di Milano,*
Italy

1. Introduction

Neuroendocrine Tumors (NETs) constitute a heterogeneous group of neoplasms which originate from neuroendocrine cells of diffuse endocrine system. They may synthesize, store, and secrete peptides and neuroamines that can cause distinct clinical syndromes. On the other hand, many are clinically silent until late presentation with mass effects (1).

Gastro-Entero-Pancreatic (GEP) NETs originate from both pancreatic islet cells or gastroenteric tissue (from diffuse neuroendocrine cells distributed throughout the gut) and are rare neoplasms, representing about 2% of all the gastrointestinal tumors. Due to their rarity, they are difficult to diagnose and the begnning of the diagnostic process is often based on the measurement of circulating markers, before planning expensive and invasive diagnostic tests (2, 3). A critical point is that the frequent late diagnosis of NETs is due to failure to identify symptoms or to establish the biochemical diagnosis; in fact 60-80% of NETs are metastatic at diagnosis. A prompt identification by the use of specific biomarkers is therefore useful to recognize these tumors (1).

Circulating tumor biomarkers can be divided into general and specific biomarkers. The neuroendocrine cells that give rise to NETs have many common features, including the synthesis of peptides, biologically inactive, that act as general markers, but have also the capacity to secrete a variety of specific biomarkers that characterize a precise biochemical function (4). Individual amines and peptide hormones are indeed specific to certain types of NETs (**Table 1**).

2. General biomarkers

There are several families of secretory proteins found in high concentrations in neuroendocrine cells and, in particular, neuroendocrine tumor cells.

They include the granins, neuron specific enolase (NSE), and pancreatic polypeptide (PP). Both chromogranin A (CgA) and NSE show increased concentration levels in many patients with NETs, but CgA is recognized as the most effective and the only general biomarker that has been extensively investigated (1-5).

Tumor Site	**Syndrome**	**Symptoms**	**Biomarkers**
Gastric (type 1 and 2)	None	Upper GI	CgA, gastrin
Gastric (type 3)	None	Upper GI	CgA
Duodenal	Zollinger-Ellison	Epigastric pain, peptic ulcer, diarrhea, GERD	CgA, gastrin (>50%), PP (35%), Somatostatin (<10%)
Ileal	Carcinoid	Diarrhea, flushing, sweating	CgA, serotonin, NKA and SP, 5HIAA
Appendix	Carcinoid	Diarrhea, flushing, sweating	CgA, serotonin, HIAA, NKA
Rectal	None	None	CgA, PYY(10%)
Meckel diverticulum	Zollinger-Ellison	Epigastric pain, peptic ulcer, diarrhea	CgA, gastrin (>50%)
Pancreas			
Insulinoma	Whipple's triad	Hypoglycemia, dizziness, sweating	CgA, insulin, pro-insulin, C-peptide
Gastrinoma	Zollinger-Ellison	Epigastric pain, peptic ulcer, diarrhea	CgA, gastrin, PP (35%)
VIP-oma	WDHA	Watery diarrhea	CgA, VIP
Glucagonoma	None	Necrolytic migratory erythema	CgA, glucagon, glycentin
Somatostatinoma	None	Mild diabetes, gallstones	CgA, somatostatin
PP-oma	None	None	CgA, PP
Non functioning	None	None	CgA, PP

CgA=Chromogranin A; 5-HIAA= 5-hydroxyindoleacetic acid; PP= Pancreatic polypeptide; VIP= vasointestinal peptide; NKA= neurokinin A; PYY= peptide YY

Table 1. Syndromes, symptoms and secretory products from GEP NETs

2.1 Granins

The chromogranin family consists of at least three different water soluble acidic glycoproteins (CgA, CgB, and secretogranin II, sometimes called chromogranin C). These proteins are 27 to 100 kDa in size and contain 10% acidic (glutamic or aspartic acid) residues, as well as multiple single and dibasic amino acid residues. All of the granins are found as major components of the soluble core of dense-core secretory granules in NE cells and are secreted from these cells in a physiologically regulated manner. Granins are major constituents of large dense-core secretory vesicles and are co-secreted with peptide hormones and amines. Electron dense or translucent secretory granules are in fact prototypical features of the neuroendocrine cells (1-6).

2.1.1 Chromogranin A (CgA)

Chromogranin A (CgA) has been claimed to be the best general neuroendocrine marker so far available. CgA is a 49 kDa monomeric, hydrophilic, acidic glycoprotein of 460 amino acid and is widely expressed in neuroendocrine cells, where it constitutes one of the most abundant components of secretory granules, and it is secreted from neuroendocrine-derived tumors including functioning and non-functioning GEP NETs, pheochromocytomas, neuroblastomas, medullary thyroid carcinomas and some pituitary tumors. CgA is secreted to the extracellular space, so it's easily detectable in the blood. CgA is co-secreted with the amines and peptides that are present in the neurosecretory granules even if it can be elevated in both functionally active and non-functional NETs. CgA seems to be a "common denominator" peptide in all the components of the diffuse neuroendocrine system (7).

The precise function of CgA remains unknown, but it is thought to be involved in the packaging and processing of neuropeptide precursor and peptide hormones. It may also play a role in the organization of the secretory granule matrix. Moreover CgA has diverse physiological interactions: CgA (or its derivatives) is an inhibitor of catecholamine, insulin, and leptin, having a role in carbohydrate and lipid metabolism; moreover it inhibits parathormone secretion; on the other hand, CgA increases glucagon and amylase release. In addition to its effects on endocrine organs, CgA also regulates reproductive functions and has a role also in the regulation of cardiovascular function: CgA elevations have been reported in essential hypertension (CgA levels correlates with the severity of hypertension) and in chronic heart failure correlating with grade of cardiac dysfunction and mortality. A role of CgA in the regulation of inflammatory response has also been described. In fact increased CgA levels correlate with serum TNF-α receptor levels in a number of inflammatory diseases including rheumatoid arthritis, inflammatory bowel disease, systemic lupus erythematosus, chronic obstructive pulmonary disease and chronic heart failure. Patients with sepsis show the highest increase of CgA; CgA positively correlates with inflammatory markers as C-reactive protein and procalcitonin. It remains to be elucidated the pathophysiological relevance of these correlations. Some authors suggest that CgA participates in a negative feedback that limits the activation of endothelial cells (1).

Circulating CgA concentrations are sensitive even if non specific markers of NETs. CgA has been reported to be more sensitive than urinary 5-hydroxyindoleacetic acid (5-HIAA) as well as than pancreatic polypeptide concentrations. The highest values were noted in ileal NETs (200 times the upper normal limit) and IN GEP-NETs associated with MEN1 (150 times the upper normal limit) while gastric type I, pituitary, and parathyroid tumors had lower values (ranging from 2 to 4 times normal). Both functioning and nonfunctioning pancreatic NETs had intermediate values (60–80 times the upper limit of normal) as did Zollinger- Ellison Syndrome (ZES), multiple endocrine neoplasia (MEN)-1, type II and III gastric entero-chromaffin-like (ECL)omas (80–100 times normal). It has also been proposed that CgA is more frequently elevated in well-differentiated tumors compared to poorly differentiated tumors of the midgut, suggesting that the loss of CgA expression in poorly differentiated neuroendocrine carcinomas indicates their incomplete or partial endocrine differentiation. In fact, poorly differentiated NE carcinomas rarely express CgA because of the rarity of large, dense-core granules. The presence of high plasma levels of CgA at diagnosis is an independent prognostic factor that indicates a reduced overall survival.

Effective treatment is often associated with decrease in CgA values. CgA correlates with tumor burden and recurrence. Measurement of CgA may help in the effective diagnosis of NET and has a major utility in predicting disease recurrence, outcome, and efficacy of therapy, so delineating the prognosis (5).

Elevated CgA can occur in normal individuals and in patients with non-NET tumors, although the levels are usually lower than in patients with NET. Less than 1% of CgA tests that are more than 20 times greater than the reference range are false positive. Levels of CgA secretion vary on a day-to-day basis in healthy subjects as well as in individuals with NETs. The mean day-to-day variation of CgA is approximately 25%. Food intake may increase CgA levels, therefore, CgA should be measured in fasting patients to ensure standardization of the results. There are conflicting results on the impact of exercise on CgA. Significant increases in CgA concentration have been reported in healthy subjects, but in patients with heart disease, long-term exercise had no impact on CgA. Finally extreme physical stress also causes CgA elevations. High-serum levels of CgA have also been demonstrated in patients with other malignancies including colon, lung, breast, liver and prostate cancer. Overall CgA has been found to be clinically informative and moderately sensitive in the majority of the studies, and more sensitive than NSE. In prostate cancer elevated CgA seems to indicate a poor prognosis; in small-cell lung carcinoma CgA levels were more frequently elevated and were also higher in cases of more extensive disease; NE differentiation occurs in 34% of primary colorectal cancer (1).

False-positive elevation of CgA may also occur in the following non-neoplastic circumstances: impaired renal function, Parkinson disease, untreated hypertension and pregnancy, steroid treatment or glucocorticoid excess, chronic atrophic gastritis (type A), treatment with proton pump inhibitors (PPI), inflammatory bowel disease, liver disease, hyperthyroidism. In renal failure CgA increases due to a decreased plasma clearance, reaching levels found in neuroendocrine neoplasia. In autoimmune chronic atrophic gastritis, elevated circulating CgA levels are caused by chronic hypergastrinemia and stimulation of ECL cell proliferation. Raised circulating CgA levels in addition to raised gastrin in atrophic gastritis, confounds the diagnosis of gastrinoma in many patients who present with dyspeptic symptoms. But the major cause of elevated CgA levels is the widespread use of PPIs and other acid suppressive medications. All PPI users, even with low dosage (10 mg/d) have elevated fasting CgA levels. The normalization of CgA levels occurs by withdrawal of PPI in 1-2 weeks (1, 10).

There is no universal standard calibration for serum or plasma chromogranin A assays. In addition, different chromogranin A assays, which use different antibodies or antibody combinations, will display different cross-reactivity with the various chromogranin A fragments. Therefore, reference intervals and individual patient results differ significantly between different chromogranin A assays and cannot be directly compared. Several commercially available radioimmunoassays (RIAs) and enzyme-linked immunosorbent assays (ELISAs) have been developed for the measurement of circulating CgA concentrations. Moreover many diagnostic laboratories use in-house assays. The three main different commercial kits are CgA-RIA CT (CIS Bio International, Gif-sur-Yvette Cedex, France), Dako CgA ELISA kit (Dako A/S, Glostrup, Denmark), and CgA EuroDiagnostica (ED) (Malmo¨, Sweden). All three assays use different standards. In the CIS kit, CgA concentration is expressed in ng/ml and normal range is < 99μg/l, while with the

Dako assay results are expressed in U/l, and normal range is within 19 U/l; with the ED kit CgA levels are expressed in nmol/l and normal range is < 41 nmol/l. Concerning plasma and serum measurement, a strong positive linear relationship has been reported between plasma and serum CgA values, indicating that CgA measurement can be undertaken in both sample types. In conclusion, because CgA concentrations are of considerable clinical relevance, substantial characterization and standardization to ensure uniform reporting are needed (1, 7, 8).

2.1.2 Other granin family peptides

The granin family comprises eight members including CgA and its derivated peptides, CgB, CgC (secretogranin II [SgII]), SgIII, SgIV, SgV, SgVI and VGF, but their value as circulating markers for endocrine tumors has not been investigated extensively extensively (1).

Several other CgA-derived peptides, resulting by posttranslational processing have been isolated from extracts of human endocrine tumors. These molecules results in a series of smaller biologically active peptides, such as pancreastatin (corresponding to CgA residues 250–301), catestatin (corresponding to CgA residues 352–372), and vasostatin I and II (corresponding to CgA residues 1–76 and 1–113, respectively). These CgA derived peptides affect secretion of other hormones, play a role in vasoconstriction, and regulate metabolism. Among them, the most clinically interesting is pancreastatin. An endoprotease, the prohormone convertase-1 (PC-1), is involved in the processing of the precursor protein chromogranin A (CGA) to a smaller peptide called pancreastatin (PST), a 49-aminoacid peptide that inhibits insulin secretion, somatostatin release, exocrine pancreatic secretion and gastric acid secretion. PST is found in human stomach- and colon extracts and in a liver metastasis of gastrinoma. Pancreastatin was used before the complete sequence of CgA had been elucidated and before there were any reliable assays that could measure the whole molecule of CgA, as an epitope for antibody production. Pancreastatin antisera were used in immunohistochemistry and RIA to assess the presence of CgA in cells and the concentration of CgA in the circulation. But pancreastatin levels do not equale to CgA concentrations in the circulation. The molecule was found to be significantly increased in patients with NETs metastasized to the liver and concentrations are proportional to the number of hepatic metastases. Monitoring of liver metastases may remain the main advantage of pancreastatin assay (2). It is interesting that pancreastatin is not increased in patients with gastric achlorhydria or hypochlorhydria. Thus, false-positives are less problematic with the pancreastatin assay. It may be a very early biomarker for liver tumor activity, even when CgA is normal (5).

CgB is the second most abundant member of the chromogranin family. Like CgA, it is a strongly acid protein containing approximately 25% acidic amino acid residues. It has 14 dibasic cleavage points but has been less well studied than CgA. Unlike CgA, CgB does not seem to have increased concentrations in patients with renal failure, in patients with atrophic gastritis, or those receiving acid-suppressing therapy. The interest to measure CgB in addition to CgA in patients with GEP NETs is therefore increased. Moreover, in tumors where CgA is not found, CgB may be increased. Such patients include those with MEN 1 and those with tumors in the duodenum or rectum. In addition, CgB is a major granin of the human adrenal medulla and may be a more sensitive marker of pheochromocytomas (2, 5).

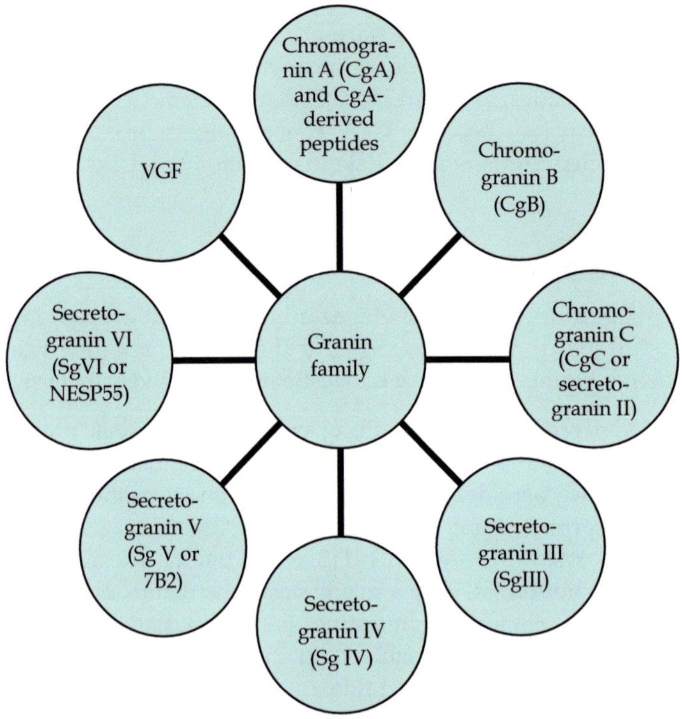

Fig. 1. The granin family and fragments of CgA. The 8 granin proteins include chromogranin A, CgB, CgC (SgII), SgIII, SgIV, 7B2 (SgV), neuroendocrine secretory protein 55 (NESP55 or SgVI), and VGF nerve growth factor–inducible (VGF).

2.2 Pancreatic polypeptide (PP)

Circulating PP is a single chain, 36-aminoacid peptide arising from the PP cells of the pancreas and is expressed in neuroendocrine cells of the gut and the pancreas. The function of PP is to self regulate pancreatic secretion activities (endocrine and exocrine), it also has effects on hepatic glycogen levels and gastrointestinal secretions.

Elevated PP concentration are found in patients with NETs, both pancreatic (20-50%) and gastrointestinal carcinoids (30-50%). Before methods for the measurements of CgA were available, PP was used as a general marker for endocrine tumors, although it is poorly specific. PP is now useful in the diagnosis and monitoring of NETs where no other general marker is raised and in PP-omas. High levels of circulating PP can also be found in diabetes, renal impairment, chronic inflammation, alcoholism and in elder patients. Its secretion is increased after a protein meal, fasting, exercise, and acute hypoglycemia and is decreased by somatostatin and intravenous glucose (2, 11).

2.3 Neuron Specific Enolase (NSE)

NSE is the neuron-specific isomer of the glycolytic enzyme 2-phospho-D-glycerate hydroxylase or enolase. This isomer is present in neurons and neuroendocrine cells and can be used as a biomarker for tumors derived from these cells. As well as CgA, NSE is a marker useful for the diagnosis and the monitoring of patients with neuroendocrine tumors (especially neuroblastoma, small cell lung cancer, less important for GEP NETs); it has other several applications, including the assessment of neuronal damage during stroke. Elevated NSE levels are indicative of poorly differentiated tumors. NSE levels seems not to be related to any secretory activity of the tumor (11, 12).

3. Specific biomarkers

In addition to general markers, there are biomarkers specific for particular GEP-NET associated syndromes. The most typical is carcinoid syndrome and the specific marker is 5-Hydroxyindole Acetic Acid. Other specific markers including insulin, gastrin, vasoactive intestinal peptide, glucagon, bradykinin, substance P, neurotensin, human chorionic gonadotropin, neuropeptide K, and neuropeptide L are each of some value in precisely defining the functionality of individual NETs (see above **Table 1**).

3.1 5-Hydroxyindole acetic acid (5-HIAA)

5-HIAA is the urinary breakdown of serotonin, which is synthesized and stored in enterochromaffin cells of the gastrointestinal tract (80% of total body serotonin content), in dense granules of platelets and in the serotoninergic neurons of the central nervous system. Serotonin is a ubiquitous tryptophan-derived biogenic amine, involved in homeostasis, vasoconstriction and neurotransmission (7).

Carcinoid syndrome is the typical clinical picture of metastatic ileal carcinoid, occurring in about 18% of patients and is characterized by flushing, diarrhea, abdominal pain; less frequent events are lacrymation, profuse sweating, telangiectasias, cardiac fibrosis, and cutaneous manifestations pellagra-like due to lack of niacin. This syndrome is caused by the massive release of serotonin, which is no longer metabolized in the liver, and other substances, such as tachykinins, prostaglandins, and bradykinins (3) (**Table 2**).

Clinical features	**(%)**	**Characteristics**	**Mediators**
Flushing	90	*Foregut* tumors: prolonged fit, red-purple, localized to face and trunk. *Midgut* tumors: quick fit, pink-red.	Serotonin, histamine, P substance, prostaglandins
Diarrhea	70	Secretory	Serotonin, histamine, VIP, prostaglandins, gastrin
Abdominal pain	40	Long lasting	Obstruction, hepatomegaly, intestinal ischemia, fibrosis
Profuse sweating	15		Serotonin, histamine
Telangiectasias	25	Face	Unknown cause
Heart disease	30 (right) 10 (left)	Valvulopathies (tricuspid valve, pulmonary valve). Right heart failure. Dyspnea	P substance, serotonin
Pellagra	5	Dermatitis	deficit of niacin

Table 2. Characteristics of carcinoid syndrome

This syndrome is typical of metastatic well-differentiated midgut NETs, even if other clinical conditions may mimic symptoms and signs (**Table 3**).

Clinical Condition	**Tests**
Carcinoid	CgA, Serotonin, 5-HIAA, PP, VIP
VIP-oma	CgA, PP, VIP
Medullary carcinoma of the thyroid	CgA, CEA, Calcitonin, Ca++ infusion, RET proto-oncogene
Pheocromocytoma	CgA, Plasma free metanephrines, urine metanephrines, VMA, Epi, Norepi, glucagon stimulation, MIBG
Diabetic autonomic neuropathy	HRV, 2hs PP glucose
Menopause	FSH
Epilepsy	EEG
Panic attack	Pentagastrin, ACTH
Mastocytosis	Plasma histamine, urine tryptase
Mitral valve prolapse	Cardiac echo

CgA=Chromogranin A; 5-HIAA= 5-hydroxyindoleacetic acid; PP= Pancreatic polypeptide; VIP= vasointestinal peptide; CEA= carcino-embryonic antigen; VMA= vanillylmandelic acid; Epi= epinephrine; Norepi= norepinephrine; MIBG= metaiodobenzylguanidine; HRV= heart rate variability; 2hs PP= 2-hour postprandial blood sugar; FSH= follicle-stimulating hormone; EEG= electroencephalography; ACTH= adrenocorticotropic hormone.

Table 3. Differential diagnosis of flushing and diagnostic tests

The 24-h measurement of 5-HIAA is a useful specific marker for serotonin-producing NETs. The overall sensitivity and specificity of urinary 5-HIAA in the presence of the carcinoid syndrome is 70 and 90%, respectively. Therefore this marker is the most frequently performed assay in the clinical setting of the carcinoid syndrome. Midgut carcinoids are most liable to produce the carcinoid syndrome with 5-HIAA elevation, thus attesting to a high specificity in this setting (approximately 75% of midgut NETs are associated with a positive urinary 5-HIAA test). Functional symptoms in NETs originating from the midgut are in fact mostly due to the secretion of 5-hydroxytryptophan (5-HTP) or serotonin. The sensitivity is lower in patients with midgut carcinoid tumors without the carcinoid syndrome and in patients with fore- and hindgut NETs due to less serotonin production from these tumors than midgut ones. Elevated 5-HIAA levels in the urine are highly suggestive of an ileal NET, although some NETs found in the lung and pancreas also secrete serotonin (7, 11).

High-performance-liquid-chromatography (HPLC) with electrochemical detection is currently recommended to measure 5-HIAA. In some laboratory automated assays or those using mass spectrometry are available.

There are false positive 5-HIAA urinary levels as well as false negative ones. Some foods contain high levels of serotonin which may increase the levels of urinary 5-HIAA and their consumption should be avoided 3 days prior to urine collection (i.e. plums, pineapples, bananas, eggplants, tomatoes, avocados, and walnuts). For this reason patients need to be on a diet free of tryptophan/serotonin-rich foods to avoid false elevations in urinary 5-

HIAA. Untreated patients with malabsorption (celiac disease, tropical sprue, Whipple disease, intestinal stasis and cystic fibrosis), may have increased tryptophan metabolites. Also certain medications may interfere with the assay: paracetamol, fluorouracil, methysergide, naproxen and caffeine may cause false positive results. On the contrary levodopa, aspirin, adrenocorticotrophic hormone (ACTH), methyldopa, and phenothiazines may give a false negative results (13). Somatostatin analogs are known to decrease levels of 5-HIAA. Moreover, patients with renal impairment and those with hemodyalisis may have falsely low 5-HIAA levels.

5-HIAA does not seem to be a useful prognostic factor in patients with carcinoid syndrome, because of the fluctuating release of serotonin in NETs of the midgut. On the other hand, several studies found high 5-HIAA levels to be an independent survival factor. Overall, in these studies, higher concentrations of urinary 5-HIAA are associated with a worse prognosis, and persistently low 5-HIAA excretion predicts more favorable survival in patients with disseminated disease. The intra-individual variation of 5-HIAA may be high. When the collection is required for the diagnosis it is useful to have two consecutive 24-hours collections and to take the mean value (7).

Serotonin plays a key role in development of peritoneal and cardiac fibrosis via activation of the 5HT2B receptor and a cascade of connective tissue growth factors. Reductions in plasma serotonin levels correlate with a decreased incidence of carcinoid heart disease (CHD). Moreover, urinary 5-HIAA excretion also correlates with the severity of CHD and prognosis in patients with carcinoid syndrome.

3.2 Insulin

Insulin is a peptide hormone composed of 51 amino acids and has a molecular weight of 5808 Da. It is produced in the islets of Langerhans in the pancreas, within the β-cells. In β-cells, insulin is synthesized from the proinsulin precursor molecule. Insulin is a hormone central in the regulation of carbohydrate and fat metabolism in the body. Since the main action of insulin is reducing blood glucose levels, by increasing glycogen synthesis and promoting storage of glucose in liver (and muscle) cells, insulin excess (such as an insulinoma) induces hypoglycemia. In patients with suspected insulinoma, the insulin and its precursors or breakdown products should be tested, even if further biochemical tests include the 72-hour fast, which is the gold standard for establishing the diagnosis of insulinoma. Insulinomas secrete proinsulin, insulin and C-peptide intermittently, and, although insulin concentrations in the circulation may often be within reference range, insulin is at most times inappropriately high for the blood glucose concentration (14).

Insulinoma is the most common secretory NET of the pancreas that produces a symptomatic clinical syndrome. More than 80% of insulinomas are benign. Insulinoma is uncommon, although it is the second most common pancreatic NET to occur in patients with MEN1 (5).

3.3 Gastrin

Gastrin is a hormone that stimulates secretion of gastric acid (HCl) by the parietal cells of the stomach and aids in gastric motility. It is released by G cells in the stomach, duodenum, and the pancreas. Gastrinoma (gastrin-producing tumor) is the second most common secretory pancreatic NET. It can rise from both cells in the duodenum and in the pancreas, with just more than half malignant at presentation. Approximately 25% to 35% of gastrinomas are associated with MEN1. Gastrinoma is the most common GEP NET associated with MEN1. Gastrinomas secrete gastrin but gastrin can circulate in numerous forms. Progastrin, gastrin 34, gastrin 17, and C-terminally extended gastrins may all circulate in high concentrations in patients with gastrinoma. In the Zollinger-Ellison syndrome, gastrin is produced at excessive levels. Normal values are generally less than 100 pg/mL (2, 5).

Gastrinoma is not the only cause of hypergastrinemia, since there are several causes for hypergastrinemia that often require numerous and expensive diagnostic investigations. Hypergastrinemia is most frequently due to hypochlorhydria and only seldom the underlying cause is gastrinoma. The most frequent condition that causes hypochlorhydria is the use of antacids or medicines that suppress stomach acid. Also autoimmune gastritis, where the immune system attacks the parietal cells leading to hypochlorhydria (low stomach acidity) is a possible cause. In this condition, hypochlorhydria results in an elevated gastrin level in an attempt to compensate for increased pH in the stomach. Eventually, all the parietal cells are lost and achlorhydria results to a loss of negative feedback on gastrin secretion. Other causes of hypergastrinemia are G-cell hyperplasia (overactivity of gastrin-producing cells in the stomach), Helicobacter pylori infection of the stomach, mucolipidosis type IV (5, 15) (**Table 4**).

HYPERGASTRINEMIA WITHOUT GASTRIC ACID HYPERSECRETION:
Atrophic gastritis (with or without pernicious anemia) Gastric cancer without involvement of the gastric antrum Therapy with H-2 blockers or proton pump inhibitors (PPIs)
HYPERGASTRINEMIA WITH GASTRIC ACID HYPERSECRETION:
Gastrinoma Antral G cell hyperplasia Duodenal ulcer Gastrojejunostomy or Billroth II Pyloric stenosis Hypercalcemia Massive bowel resection Chronic renal impairment

Table 4. Conditions associated with hypergastrinemia

3.4 VIP

Vasoactive intestinal peptide (VIP) is a peptide hormone containing 28-amino acid residues. It is produced in many areas of the human body including the gut, pancreas and suprachiasmatic nuclei of the hypothalamus in the brain.

In normal physiology VIP acts as a neuromodulator and not as an hormone, since it circulates in low quantity even an increase of about 20-50% of normal reference range is significant. VIP is released from neurons, peripheral ganglia, throughout the GI tract, in the urogenital system, respiratory tract and blood vessels. VIP has several effects on the digestive system:

it relaxes the lower esophageal sphincter ,the fundic smooth muscle and suppress gastric acid secretion. These effects work together to increase motility. Like secretin, it stimulates secretion of water and bicarbonate and stimulates secretion of chloride and water from large intestine; in small intestine inhibits absorption and the contractile effect of CCK. Moreover it enhances the release of insulin and glucagon. VIP has also significant effects on the cardiovascular system. It causes coronary vasodilation as well as it has a positive inotropic and chronotropic effect. VIP helps to regulate prolactin secretion (2).

VIPoma is much less common that insulinoma and gastrinoma with an incidence of approximately 0.02 per 100,000 per year. VIPoma is characterized by watery diarrhea, hypokalemia and achlorhydria (WDHA syndrome or pancreatic cholera syndrome, or also called Verner Morrison syndrome). Due to VIP effects as a potent stimulator of intestinal secretion and inhibitor of gastric acid secretion, the massive amounts of secreted VIP cause profound and chronic **w**atery **d**iarrhea (fasting stool volume > 750 to 1000 mL/day) and resultant dehydration, **h**ypokalemia, **a**chlorhydria (hence WDHA-syndrome), acidosis, vasodilation (flushing and hypotension), hypercalcemia and hyperglycemia. The watery diarrhea may be intermittent at the onset , but it may rapidly escalate and reach a volume of 15-20L per day, causing profound alteration in fluids and electrolytes control. Hypokalemic acidosis is due to bicarbonate and potassium loss across the bowel mucosa; it may provoke asthenia and tetanic contraction. Gastric achlorhydria occurs only in 50% of patients, while hypochlorhydria is usually present. Abdominal pain and weight loss are also common features. Other signs are hypercalcemia, related to VIP direct action on bone metabolism, and flushes that may cause some confusion with classical midgut carcinoid syndrome (5) (see above, **Table 3**).

The majority of VIPomas occurs in the pancreas, while about 10-15% arises in the ganglionic chain and most common in the adrenal medulla. In children, besides, VIP-producing tumors may occur in ganglioneuroma and neuroblastoma. About 50-60% of VIP-secreting tumors are malignant and present hepatic involvement. It may arise in contest of MEN1 syndrome (2).

3.5 Glucagon

Glucagon is a hormone secreted by alpha cells (α-cells) of the islets of Langerhans of the pancreas and from the L cells in the intestinal mucosa. Glucagon is a 29-amino acid polypeptide and its main action is to raise blood glucose levels. From these two sites, proglucagon is processed differently. In the pancreas, proglucagon is processed to produce glucagon, glycentin-related peptide, intervening peptide, and the major glucagon fragment. Intestinal proglucagon undergoes alternative posttranslational processing that generates glycentin, sometimes referred to as gut glucagon, glucagon-like peptide 1 (GLP1), and glucagon-like peptide 2 (GLP2) (2).

Plasma glucagon is a specific marker for Glucagonoma. Glucagonoma occurs at approximately the same frequency as VIPoma. Circulating glucagon concentrations are typically more than 5-fold higher than the reference range. Both pancreatic glucagon and glycentin are measured in high concentrations. Considering the importance of glucagon in the control of blood glucose, one would expect a glucagon-secreting tumor to produce a profound syndrome. However this is not the case and glucagonoma usually presents late with extensive metastatic spread, mild diabetes, and a characteristic rash (necrolytic migratory erythema) (5).

Increased secretion of glucagon is also caused by other causes, like decreased plasma glucose (indirectly), increased catecholamines - norepinephrine and epinephrine, increased plasma amino acids (to protect from hypoglycemia if an all-protein meal is consumed), sympathetic nervous system, acetylcholine, cholecystokinin. Decreased secretion of glucagon is caused by somatostatin, insulin, increased free fatty acids and keto acids into the blood, increased urea production (16).

3.6 Somatostatin

Somatostatin is a peptide hormone that regulates the endocrine system and affects neurotransmission and cell proliferation. Somatostatin is classified as an inhibitory hormone, that exerts its effects mainly on anterior pituitary, by inhibiting the release of GH, opposing the effects of Growth Hormone-Releasing Hormone (GHRH), and inhibiting the release of thyroid-stimulating hormone (TSH) and on gastrointestinal system, by suppressing the release of other gastrointestinal and pancreatic hormones, decreasing gastric emptying, and reducing smooth muscle contractions and blood flow within the intestine (2).

Pancreatic somatostatinoma is a tumor of the delta cells of the endocrine pancreas that produces somatostatin. It is uncommon and symptoms are vague, thus diagnosis is frequently delayed. Clinical syndrome is characterized by a triad of : mild diabetes mellitus, steatorrhea and gallstones. Also hypochlorhydria can be associated. Patients may present with clinical endocrine syndrome due to elevated somatostatin that can cause diabetes mellitus, by inhibiting insulin secretion, steatorrhea by inhibiting cholecystokinin and secretin, gallstones by inhibiting cholecystokinin which normally induce gallbladder myocytes contraction, and hypochlorhydria caused by inhibiting gastrin, which normally stimulates acid secretion. However, more frequently patients present with symptoms related with tumor bulk. In presence of a somatostatinoma circulating somatostatin concentrations may be more than 100 times the reference range (2, 5).

3.7 Other circulating markers

3.7.1 Corticotropin-releasing hormone (CRH)

Corticotropin-releasing hormone, a 41-amino acid peptide derived from a 191-amino acid preprohormone, acts as hormone and neurotransmitter in the stimulation of pituitary synthesis of ACTH in stress response. In normal physiology CRH is produced by parvocellular neuroendocrine cells (contained within the paraventricular nucleus of hypothalamus).

Ectopic CRH production is rare, it may occur in patients with medullary thyroid carcinoma (about 33%) and pheochromocytoma (19%), carcinoid (5%) and small cell lung carcinoma (about 10 %) and prostate cancer (17). The main clinical feature is Cushing 's syndrome; levels of cortisol are elevated (>900 nmol/l) as ACTH, DHEA-S. Overnight administration of dexamethasone doesn't suppress cortisol secretion.

3.7.2 Growth-hormone-releasing-hormone (GHRH)

Growth-hormone-releasing-hormone (GHRH) is a 44-amino acid hormone released from neurosecretory nerve terminals of the arcuate neurons, and is carried by the hypothalamic-hypophyseal portal system to anterior pituitary gland, where stimulates growth hormone (GH) secretion. Hypothalamic tumors, including hamartomas, choristomas, gliomas, and gangliocytomas, may produce excessive GHRH with subsequent GH hypersecretion and resultant acromegaly. Peripheral GHRH levels are not elevated in patients with hypothalamic GHRH-secreting tumors, supporting the notion that excess eutopic hypothalamic GHRH secretion into the hypophyseal portal system does not appreciably enter the systemic circulation. Excessive ectopic peripheral production of GHRH is present in several tumors, including carcinoid tumors, pancreatic cell tumors, small-cell lung cancers, adrenal adenomas, and pheochromocytomas, which have been reported to secrete GHRH. In these cases, peripheral GHRH levels are elevated even if acromegaly in these patients, is uncommon. For these reasons measuring GHRH plasma levels provides a precise and cost-effective test for the diagnosis of ectopic acromegaly. Elevated circulating GHRH levels, a normal or small-size pituitary gland, or clinical and biochemical features of other tumors known to be associated with extra-pituitary acromegaly, are all indications for extra-pituitary production of GHRH (18).

3.7.3 Calcitonin

Calcitonin is a 32-amino acid peptide released, in normal physiology, only in non-follicular C-cells of the thyroid . It is produced as a 136-amino acid precursor (pro-calcitonin) and processed in secretory granules to the active form. The synthesis and release of calcitonin are closely related to calcium serum levels. Calcitonin is raised in medullary thyroid cancer, where concentration may be thousands-fold the reference range. Medullary thyroid cancers frequently arise as part of multiple endocrine neoplasia type 2 (MEN2) syndrome. Calcitonin may also be raised in some pancreatic neuroendocrine tumor, especially those that are multi-hormone producing and bronchial carcinoid. Usually ectopic-produced calcitonin is a large molecule without biochemical activity (2).

4. Provocative tests

4.1 Insulinoma: 72-hour fast

NETs secreting insulin are termed insulinomas and are almost exclusively intrapancreatic in nature. Insulinomas secrete proinsulin, insulin and C-peptide intermittently, and, although insulin concentrations in the circulation may often be within reference range, insulin is at most times inappropriately high for the blood glucose concentration.

The diagnosis is suggested in the presence of the Whipple's triad: symptoms of hypoglycemia, glucose < 2.5 mmol/l (45 mg/dl) and relief of symptoms with administration of glucose. Hypoglycemia-induced clinical signs are classically present in the early morning pre-prandial phase or maybe exercise-induced. The typical signs are due to activation of adrenergic nervous system (palpations, sweating pallor, anxiety) and neuroglycopenia (personality changes, and loss of consciousness). The latter symptom reflects both the severity and duration of hypoglycemia. Although these symptoms are profound, they may be intermittent and diagnosis is not always straightforward. The 72-hour fast is the gold standard for diagnosing insulinoma and it attests autonomous insulin secretion and the failure of appropriate insulin suppression in the presence of hypoglycemia. In fact, a carefully supervised 72-hour starvation usually precipitates hypoglycemia within the first 36 to 48 hours. A 72-hour period is universally recognized as the most appropriate duration although some groups have proposed a shorter fast of 48 h. Symptoms appear within 12 h for one third of patients, 80% within 24 h, 90% with 48 h and approaching 100% within 72 h. Absolute values of glucose and insulin are the most important variables and any measurable insulin is abnormal when blood glucose drops to 2.5 mol/l (45 mg/dl). The patient should be monitored in a supervised environment and fasting should be accompanied by an intravenous line. Absolute blood (venous) determinations should be performed at least 2–4 times per day and bedside measurements can be used in the presence of clinical symptoms to determine if more definitive measurements should be made. Blood should also be drawn for insulin measurement concurrently with glucose estimations, and assay for insulin and C-peptide when the hypoglycemia is confirmed. The differential diagnosis is insulin abuse (known insulin-requiring diabetes or factitious hypoglycemia): it can be detected when insulin is increased but not pro-insulin or C-peptide, so the measurement of increased pro-insulin or C-peptide secures the diagnosis of insulinoma. On rare occasions the abuse of sulphonylureas and related insulin secretagogues result in a clinical picture similar to patients with insulinoma and may be diagnosed only by a positive drug screen. Even patients on regular therapy with oral hypoglycemic medications in the setting of renal impairment may show symptoms that mimic insulinoma (5, 7).

4.2 Gastrinoma: Secretin test

Gastrinoma is the second most common secretory pancreatic NET with just more than half malignant at presentation. Gastrinoma is the most common GEP NET associated with MEN1, with approximately 25-35%of gastrinomas being associated with MEN1. Gastrinomas may be found in the duodenum (50-70%) and less commonly in the pancreas (20-40%) and secrete excess of gastrin, leading to ulceration in the stomach, duodenum and the small intestine. Hydrochloric acid (HCl) also causes hyperperistalsis and inhibits the activity of lipase causing severe diarrhea. The clinical syndrome is therefore characterized by the classical triad of gastric acid hypersecretion, severe peptic ulceration, and non-beta cell islet tumor of pancreas (gastrinoma) and this is called Zollinger Ellison syndrome (ZES). Despite a clear clinical syndrome, the primary gastrinoma may be often smaller than can be visualized by any current radiological method. Therefore, circulating gastrin remains a useful tool for diagnosis. The diagnosis of ZES can be established by the demonstration of elevated fasting serum gastrin (FSG) in the presence of low gastric pH (<5.0). In fact, in the presence of gastric acid (pH<5.0), a serum gastrin value greater than 1000 pg/mL is virtually diagnostic of the disorder. However, about two-thirds of patients with the Zollinger-Ellison syndrome have serum gastrin concentrations less than 10 times the upper limit of normal (generally between 150 and 1000 pg/mL), so FSG alone is not adequate for a conclusive diagnosis of ZES. Moreover hypergastrinemia can be seen in patients with achlorhydria associated with chronic atrophic fundus gastritis (e.g., pernicious anemia), proton pump inhibitor drugs and in other conditions with hyperchlorhydria (e.g., Helicobacter pylori infection, gastric outlet obstruction, renal failure, antral G cell syndromes, short bowel syndrome, retained antrum) (see above **Table 4**) (2).

The secretin stimulation test can differentiate patients with gastrinomas from those with hypergastrinemia of different etiologies and identify those patients with gastrinoma and only mild hypergastrinemia (**Figure 2**). Secretin is normally secreted by duodenal S-cells in response to a low luminal pH following food-stimulated acid secretion. Its primary action is to cause the release of bicarbonate rich pancreatic juice from pancreatic acinar cells, thus neutralizing the acidic juice delivered from the stomach. Under physiological conditions, secretin decreases antral gastrin secretion. However in presence of a gastrinoma, secretin stimulates the release of stored gastrin by gastrinoma cells, and therefore most patients with these tumors have a dramatic rise in serum gastrin in response to a secretin infusion. In contrast, normal gastric G cells are inhibited by secretin, and therefore serum gastrin concentrations do not rise in patients with other causes of hypergastrinemia. The secretin stimulation test is performed by administering 2 U of secretin/kg body weight intravenously over one minute; a baseline serum gastrin is measured twice before the secretin is administered and 2, 5, 10, 15, and 20 minutes later. Several criteria have been proposed to define a positive test; the most commonly accepted one is a rise in serum gastrin by 200 pg/mL (95 pmol/L) or more, which is diagnostic for the presence of gastrinoma in more than 90% of cases. The use of this test has recently been re-evaluated, suggesting a lower cut-off (a rise >120 pg/mL in serum gastrin concentration) to define a positive test, thus obtaining an increase in the sensitivity (94%) without loss of specificity (100%) (7, 15).

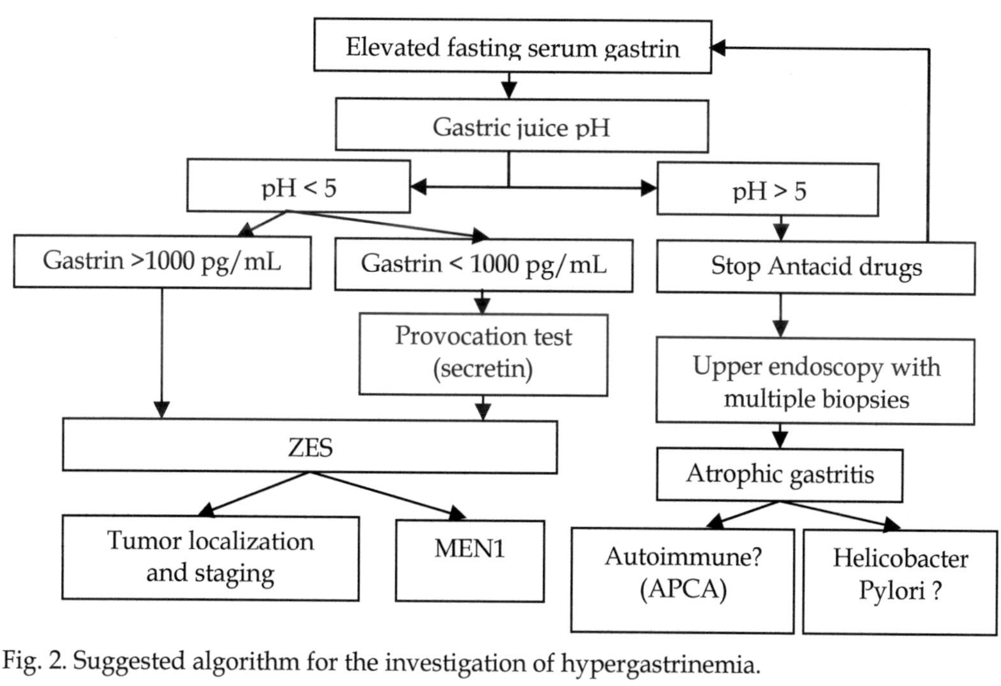

Fig. 2. Suggested algorithm for the investigation of hypergastrinemia.

Another critical point regarding secretin test is to establish whether the the same diagnostic operative characteristics of the test remains unchanged even during treatment with inhibitors of acid secretion. In fact the standard secretin test was performed with patients off antacids and anticholinergics for at least 12 hours and H2 antagonists and proton pump inhibitors were not available at the time the test was described. However, patients with severe ZES can develop complications (such as acute bleeding and perforation) if acid suppression is discontinued. Thus, discontinuation of acid suppression should be performed cautiously. While the accuracy of the test in patients taking proton pump inhibitors (PPIs) has not been well established, some authors suggest that PPIs do not interfere with the interpretation of the secretin stimulation test and that PPIs do not need to be discontinued. However, the leading experts suggest PPIs should be discontinued for one-two weeks (1, 7, 10).

The secretin stimulation test has also been shown to be a valuable predictor of recurrence of gastrinoma following surgery (15).

4.3 Other provocative tests for gastrinoma

In addition to the secretin test, several other stimulation tests have been developed to attempt to differentiate between neoplastic and non-neoplastic causes of hypergastrinemia. These include calcium, meal and glucagon stimulation tests.

4.3.1 Calcium stimulation test

The calcium provocation test is based on the principle that calcium administration stimulates the release of stored gastrin from gastrinoma cells, as well as for secretin test. Serum gastrin concentrations are measured at 0, 30, 60, 90, 120, 150, 180 minutes intervals during an intravenous infusion of 10% calcium gluconate (5 mg/kg body weight over 3 h). More than 80% of gastrinoma patients show an increase in serum gastrin of >200 pg/mL within the third hour of calcium infusion, usually with a positive response at 120 to 180 min. The sensitivity of this test is low (about 43%), thus it can't replace the secretin test, but it could be used in patients with an high clinical suspicion of ZES and a negative secretin test (15).

4.3.2 Meal stimulation test

The physiological response to a standard test meal (of two eggs and toast) is an increase in plasma gastrin of up to two to threefold. Patients with ZES demonstrate no or only a very minimal increase in serum gastrin concentration after ingestion of such a protein rich test meal, whereas patients with other causes of hypergastrinemia show a more pronounced increase in serum gastrin following the same protein test meal. However, data on these results seems to be conflicting and a significant overlap in patients with ZES and with other antral syndromes is observed, thus the meal stimulation test for investigation of the cause of hypergastrinemia is not currently recommended (15).

4.3.3 Glucagon stimulation test

Glucagon stimulation test consists in a rise in serum gastrin concentration following the administration of glucagon to patients with ZES, but a paradoxical fall in serum gastrin concentrations in patients with pernicious anemia. This test has not been widely evaluated; however, further studies are required to determine the overall accuracy of the glucagon stimulation test (15).

5. Conclusions

Numerous biochemical markers have been identified in association with GEP-NETs, but few have the specificity or predictive value of CgA or urinary 5-HIAA, and their measurement is complex. Recent studies have proposed that alkaline phosphatase and neurokinin A are better predictors of survival in metastatic NETs than CgA but additional rigorous data to support this assertion are required.

Circulating biomarkers offer a useful diagnostic tool in conjunction with radiology and tissue pathology for NETs. However, these biomarkers are more reliable when used to monitor disease progression, response to treatment, and for early detection of recurrence after treatment.

6. References

[1] Modlin IM, Gustafsson BI, Moss SF, Pavel M, Tsolakis AV, Kidd M. Chromogranin A-biological function and clinical utility in neuro endocrine tumor disease. Ann Surg Oncol. 2010;17:2427-43.

[2] Ardill JE. Circulating markers for endocrine tumors of the gastroenteropancreatic tract. Ann Clin Biochem. 2008;45:539-59.

[3] Massironi S, Sciola V, Peracchi M, Ciafardini C, Spampatti MP, Conte D. Neuroendocrine tumors of the gastro-entero-pancreatic system. World J Gastroenterol. 2008:21;14:5377-84.

[4] Schott M, Kloeppel G, Raffel A, Saleh A, Knoefel WT, Sherbaum WA. Neuroendocrine Neoplasms of the gastrointestinal tract. Dtsch Arztebl Int 2011; 108: 305-12

[5] Ardill JE, O'Dorisio TM. Circulating biomarkers in neuroendocrine tumors of the enteropancreatic tract: application to diagnosis, monitoring disease, and as prognostic indicators. Endocrinol Metab Clin North Am. 2010;39:777-90.

[6] Conlon JM. Granin-derived peptides as diagnostic and prognostic markers for endocrine tumors. Regul Pept. 2010;165:5-11.

[7] O'Toole D, Grossman A, Gross D, Delle Fave G, Barkmanova J, O'Connor J, Pape UF, Plöckinger U; Mallorca Consensus Conference participants; European Neuroendocrine Tumor Society. ENETS Consensus Guidelines for the Standards of Care in Neuroendocrine Tumors: biochemical markers. Neuroendocrinology. 2009;90:194-202.

[8] Lawrence B, Gustafsson BI, Kidd M, Pavel M, Svejda B, Modlin IM. The clinical relevance of chromogranin A as a biomarker for gastroenteropancreatic neuroendocrine tumors. Endocrinol Metab Clin North Am. 2011;40:111-34.

[9] Donica H, Malecha-Jędraszek A, Strosławska E, Burska A, Szubstarski F. Significance of plasma chromogranin A determination in neuroendocrine tumour (NET) diagnosis. Folia Histochem Cytobiol. 2010;48:603-10.

[10] Vezzosi D, Walter T, Laplanche A, Raoul JL, Dromain C, Ruszniewski P, d'Herbomez M, Guigay J, Mitry E, Cadiot G, Leboulleux S, Lombard-Bohas C, Borson-Chazot F,

Ducreux M, Baudin E. Chromogranin A measurement in metastatic well-differentiated gastroenteropancreatic neuroendocrine carcinoma: screening for false positives and a prospective follow-up study. Int J Biol Markers. 2011;26:94-101.

[11] Vinik AI, Gonzales MR. New and emerging syndromes due to neuroendocrine tumors. Endocrinol Metab Clin North Am. 2011;40:19-63.

[12] Yao JC, Pavel M, Phan AT, Kulke MH, Hoosen S, St Peter J, Cherfi A, Oberg KE. Chromogranin A and Neuron-Specific Enolase as Prognostic Markers in Patients with Advanced pNET Treated with Everolimus. J Clin Endocrinol Metab. 2011 Oct 12. [Epub ahead of print]

[13] Ramage JK, Ahmed A, Ardill J, Bax N, Breen DJ, Caplin ME, Corrie P, Davar J, Davies AH, Lewington V, Meyer T, Newell-Price J, Poston G, Reed N, Rockall A, Steward W, Thakker RV, Toubanakis C, Valle J, Verbeke C, Grossman AB. Guidelines for the management of gastroenteropancreatic neuroendocrine (including carcinoid) tumours (NETs). Gut. 2011 Nov 3. [Epub ahead of print]

[14] Guettier JM, Gorden P. Insulin secretion and insulin-producing tumors. Expert Rev Endocrinol Metab. 2010;5:217-227.

[15] Murugesan SV, Varro A, Pritchard DM. Review article: Strategies to determine whether hypergastrinaemia is due to Zollinger-Ellison syndrome rather than a more common benign cause. Aliment Pharmacol Ther. 2009;29:1055-68.

[16] Van Beek AP, de Haas ER, van Vloten WA, Lips CJ, Roijers JF, Canninga-van Dijk MR. The glucagonoma syndrome and necrolytic migratory erythema: a clinical review. Eur J Endocrinol 2004; 151:531-7.

[17] Shahani S, Nudelman R. Ectopic corticotropin-releasing-hormone (CRH) syndrome from metastatic small cell carcinoma: a case report and review of literature. Diagn Path 2010;5:56

[18] Doga M, Bonadonna S, Burattin A, Giustina A. Ectopic secretion of growth hormone-releasing hormone (GHRH) in neuroendocrine tumors: relevant clinical aspects. Ann Oncol 2001;12 Suppl 2:S89-94.

4

The Diagnosis and Management of Neuroendocrine Carcinoma of Unknown Primary

Jennifer Keiser, Emily Bergsland and Eric Nakakura
University of California San Francisco
UCSF Helen Diller
Family Comprehensive Center
USA

1. Introduction

In 1907, the pathologist Siegfried Oberndorfer first coined the term "carcinoid" to describe neoplasms located in the submucosa of the ileum (Oberndorfer 1907). These small intestinal neoplasms were typically small and often multifocal. Their borders were well circumscribed. Although he initially erroneously asserted that carcinoid tumors did not metastasize, he later recognized their malignant potential.

One hundred years after Oberndorfer's initial description of carcinoid tumors, the preferred term for these neoplasms is neuroendocrine tumors (NETs). Compared with other neoplasms, NETs are rare. However, the incidence of NETs is increasing, occurring in 5.25 individuals per 100,000 persons per year in the United States (Yao, Hassan et al. 2008). Neuroendocrine tumors most commonly arise from the gastrointestinal (GI) tract and bronchopulmonary (BP) tree. Histologically, NETs vary from well differentiated to poorly differentiated and are characterized by expression of neuroendocrine markers like chromogranin A and synaptophysin. Uptake of tracer using somatostatin receptor scintigraphy is also common in well differentiated tumors.

Hormone production occurs in a minority of patients, but can cause a range of clinical syndromes, including: hypoglycemia (insulin), recurrent ulcers/diarrhea (gastrin), glucose intolerance (glucagon), watery diarrhea (vasointestinal peptide), and diarrhea, flushing, palpitations, right-sided heart valve dysfunction (serotonin). Poorly differentiated NETs are rare but can arise in nearly any location. They are associated with a poor prognosis and have a high predilection for metastases. As such, systemic chemotherapy (with a small cell lung cancer regimen) is the mainstay of therapy. Treatment for localized well differentiated tumors is surgical. Patients with advanced disease may benefit from treatment to control hormone-mediated symptoms and/or disease progression. Treatment options are evolving and include somatostatin analogs, liver-directed approaches, systemic chemotherapy, peptide receptor radionuclide therapy, interferon, and newer targeted agents (e.g. sunitinib and everolimus). The recent approval of everolimus and sunitinib in pancreatic NET specifically highlights the importance of identifying the primary site. Despite extensive evaluation, some patients are diagnosed with neuroendocrine carcinoma of unknown primary, presenting a major therapeutic challenge in the face of therapies that are increasingly disease- and site-specific.

2. Epidemiology

Patients with neuroendocrine carcinoma of unknown primary present unique clinical challenges. In a recent epidemiological study, a primary tumor site was not identified in up to 4,752 (13%) of 35,618 patients with NETs (Yao, Hassan et al. 2008).

3. Diagnostic methods used to identify the primary site

Currently, there are no clear recommendations for how best to identify the primary site in patients with advanced neuroendocrine carcinoma and an elusive primary site.

3.1 Rationale for identifying the primary site

The value of identifying the primary site depends largely on the tumor's differentiation and grade. Recognizing the fact that randomized trials are lacking, patients with advanced extra-pulmonary poorly differentiated or high grade (e.g. small or large cell) NETs are typically treated with a small cell lung cancer chemotherapy regimen. In contrast, identification of the primary site in patients with well differentiated (low and intermediate grade) NETs may directly influence treatment decisions and prognosis. Well differentiated NETs of the midgut are often associated with symptoms consistent with traditional carcinoid syndrome and may cause bleeding and obstruction from the primary tumor and regional adenopaty/fibrosis but tend to be relatively indolent. In contrast, rectal tumors do not typically cause hormone-mediated symptoms.

Some systemic treatments have selective use in NETs of known primary sites. Octreotide has been proven to improve outcomes in midgut carcinoids (Rinke, Muller et al. 2009), whereas the molecularly targeted agents sunitinib and everolimus are indicated for treatment of pancreatic NETs specifically (Raymond, Dahan et al. 2011; Yao, Shah et al. 2011). Furthermore, pancreatic NETs tend to be more sensitive to chemotherapy than carcinoids (Nakakura, Venook et al. 2007). Within carcinoid tumors, emerging data suggests that tumors of bronchial and thymic origin may be particular sensitive to temozolomide (Ekeblad, Sundin et al. 2007). Therefore, identification of the primary site may assist in prioritizing systemic treatment options and may shed light on the role of surgical intervention in a given patient (especially in the setting of resectable metastatic disease).

3.2 Methods for identifying the primary site

Imaging identifies most pancreatic NET primaries. In a recent study, computed tomography (CT) identified the majority of pancreatic NETs (84% [n=231]) (Khashab, Yong et al. 2011). This sensitivity was greater in nonfunctional pancreatic NETs (92% [n=173]). In the same study, 56 patients had combined CT and endoscopic ultrasound (EUS) imaging; EUS detected 91% [n=22] of pancreatic NETs (i.e., insulinomas) not identified on CT. Therefore, as most pancreatic NET primaries are found with CT, EUS, or hormone marker tests, the pancreas is unlikely to account for a large fraction of NETs of unknown primary once the appropriate work-up has been done.

Various diagnostic methods have been explored for detecting the primary site in the context of nonpancreatic, well differentiated NETs , which typically arise in the foregut, midgut or hindgut (i.e., carcinoid tumors). Published studies focusing on the diagnostic work-up are almost always limited by a small sample size. In particular, CT, somatostatin receptor scintigraphy , enteroclysis, capsule endoscopy, and magnetic resonance imaging enteroclysis have all been found to have some utility for identifying the primary tumor (Picus, Glazer et al. 1984; Sugimoto, Lorelius et al. 1995; Bader, Semelka et al. 2001; van Tuyl, Kuipers et al. 2004; Johanssen, Boivin et al. 2006). Recently, the sensitivity of diagnostic methods for locating primary tumors in a larger number of patients with well differentiated NET liver metastases was reported by Wang et al. (Wang, Parekh et al. 2010). Computed tomography (35% [n=78]) and somatostatin receptor scintigraphy (26% [n=42]) were not sensitive in detecting the primary sites. For patients with colonic NETs, colonoscopy detected most primary tumors (87% [n=15]).

In the study by Wang et al., 15 patients with NET liver metastases and unknown primary tumor underwent surgical exploration, 7 of which were laparoscopic. The primary tumor was located in most (87%) patients (Wang, Parekh et al. 2010). All identified tumors were in the small intestine. They were small in diameter (1.4 cm), and more than half (54%) were mutifocal. Another study also found that surgical exploration successfully localized and resected occult primary NETs in 17 of 22 (77%) patients (Boudreaux, Putty et al. 2005). Based on these data, for patients with well differentiated (low and intermediate grade) unknown primary tumors and NET liver metastases, a multidisciplinary team assessment for possible surgical exploration and resection of occult primary tumors should be considered. Before surgery, a CT scan, somatostatin receptor scintigraphy, and upper/lower endoscopy should be done (Wang, Parekh et al. 2010). EUS may be of value in identifying the location of an insulinoma (Khashab, Yong et al. 2011).

Immunohistochemical analyses using various markers are also emerging as potentially powerful tools for identification of the primary site for NETs. Expression of PAX8 or ISL1 is suggestive of a pancreatic primary tumor (Schmitt, Riniker et al. 2008; Haynes, Sangoi et al. 2011). Although CK7 and CK20 have been reported to be specific for BP- and GI-NETs, respectively (Cai, Banner et al. 2001), these findings were not corroborated by a larger study (Chu, Wu et al. 2000). TTF expression appears to be specific for BP-NETs (Agoff, Lamps et al. 2000; Oliveira, Tazelaar et al. 2001; Du, Goldstraw et al. 2004; Saqi, Alexis et al. 2005; Lin, Saad et al. 2007; Srivastava and Hornick 2009); however, its sensitivity is low and variable (Matoso, Singh et al. 2009). CDX2 is specific for GI-NETs, but it also has low and variable sensitivity and is not a good marker for pancreatic NETs (Saqi, Alexis et al. 2005; Lin, Saad et al. 2007; Srivastava and Hornick 2009). NKX2.2 is a highly sensitive and specific marker for GI-NETs, including NETs of the stomach, duodenum, ampulla of Vater, pancreas, ileum, and colon (Wang, Gallego-Arteche et al. 2009; Wang, Iezza et al. 2010). In the future, use of a panel of markers may be particularly informative (Srivastava and Hornick 2009).

Chromosomal abnormality and molecular gene profiling may have an increasing role in identifying tumor type. Jiao et al. recently reported that mutations of DAXX/ATRX, MEN1, and mTOR pathway genes are frequent in pancreatic NETs (Jiao, Shi et al. 2011).

Cunningham et al. suggest that chromosome 18 aberrations are common in both sporadic and familial ileal NETs (Cunningham, Diaz de Stahl et al. 2011). Recently, Erlander et al. recently reported on the use of a 92-gene real-time PCR assay for tumor classification used to compare the gene expression profile of an unknown sample to that of known tumors in a reference database (Erlander, Ma et al. 2011). This reference database includes NETs, such as small intestinal, BP, and pancreatic NETs. While these advances related to chromosome and gene profiling hold promise for the identification of unknown primary NETs, additional work is needed before these techniques can become standard of care.

4. Treatment and outcome

Tumor grade is of paramount importance in determining the treatment and outcome for patients with neuroendocrine carcinoma of unknown primary (Stoyianni, Pentheroudakis et al. 2011). As such, a precise determination of grade is essential. Additional tissue should be obtained if the initial sample is inadequate. Current data support that measures of proliferation rate are critical in determining grade (i.e., Ki67 index and mitotic counts). Therefore, grade is a standard feature of pathology reports describing NETs and forms the basis of the most recent NET pathology guidelines (Klimstra, Modlin et al. 2010).

4.1 Treatment of well differentiated (low and intermediate grade) unknown primary NETs

For patients with well differentiated (low and intermediate grade) NET liver metastases and an unknown primary tumor, a multidisciplinary evaluation for possible surgical exploration and resection of occult primary tumors should be considered. Interestingly, Dr. Oberndorfer's initial description of carcinoids included 6 patients with tumors arising from the ileum (Oberndorfer 1907). Over 100 years later, the jejunum/ileum remains one of the most common sites from which GI-NETs arise (Modlin, Shapiro et al. 2004). Despite their small size, NETs of the small intestine cause a characteristic fibrosis of the mesentery, leading to bowel obstruction, ischemia, or perforation in approximately one-third of patients (Makridis, Oberg et al. 1990; Boudreaux, Putty et al. 2005). Thus, the accepted standard of treatment for locoregional disease is resection of the small intestinal primary tumor and regional lymph nodes/fibrosis.

For a limited number of patients with liver metastases, hepatic resection appears to improve survival (Chen, Hardacre et al. 1998; Norton, Fraker et al. 2006). If complete resection of metastases is feasible, this should be considered. However, most patients are not candidates for liver resection because of extensive disease. For these patients, resection of the primary tumor could be beneficial. Two studies reported that resection of the midgut carcinoid primary tumor may be associated with improved outcome, even in the setting of unresectable liver metastases (Hellman, Lundstrom et al. 2002; Givi, Pommier et al. 2006). For carefully selected patients with unresectable NET liver metastases, some recommend that the primary tumor be localized and resected, even in asymptomatic patients (Boudreaux, Putty et al. 2005; Givi, Pommier et al. 2006; Wang, Parekh et al. 2010).

If surgery is not deemed prudent, patients with unknown primaries should be treated similarly as if they have advanced well differentiated NETs, assuming a pancreatic primary has been excluded (Nakakura, Venook et al. 2007; Stoyianni, Pentheroudakis et al. 2011). In particular, treatment with somatostatin receptor analog therapy (i.e., octreotide) should be considered, especially for those with carcinoid syndrome. The results from the PROMID study suggest that octreotide has an antitumor effect in midgut carcinoids in addition to controlling hormone-mediated symptoms--the indication for which it has FDA approval (Rinke, Muller et al. 2009). In this placebo-controlled, double-blind, prospective study, patients treated with octreotide had a 14.3 month median time to progression compared to 6 months in the placebo group (Rinke, Muller et al. 2009). Of note, the primary site was unknown in 21 patients, and these patients were considered eligible for the study; however, NETs of the lung, pancreas, and other sites were excluded. Importantly, the optimal timing of treatment in patients with nonfunctional tumors (i.e., at diagnosis or after documented disease progression) and the value specifically in unknown primary tumors remains somewhat uncertain.

Unfortunately, aside from octreotide, systemic treatment options are extremely limited for advanced, nonpancreatic, well differentiated NETs (Chan and Kulke 2011; Strosberg, Cheema et al. 2011). Interferon is associated with stability and biochemical control in some cases, but radiographic responses are rare. There are little data to support cytotoxic chemotherapy in well differentiated NETs, although streptozotocin-based regimens may have limited activity at the expense of toxicity (Nakakura, Venook et al. 2007). Temozolamide-based regimens have emerged as potentially active in pancreatic and poorly differentiated NETs (Strosberg, Fine et al. 2011; Welin, Sorbye et al. 2011). Nevertheless, many believe that cytotoxic chemotherapy should be an option for patients who have failed other therapies, recognizing that no standard regimen exists (Boudreaux, Klimstra et al. 2010). Additional treatments are needed, and enrollment on clinical trials is encouraged.

Emerging data suggest that vascular endothelial growth factor (VEGF) and mTOR are valid targets for therapy in pancreatic NETs, as evidenced by the recent approval of sunitinib and everolimus in this disease (Raymond, Dahan et al. 2011; Yao, Shah et al. 2011). The value of these agents in well differentiated NETs arising outside of the pancreas is uncertain. In the RADIANT-2 study, patients with progressive nonpancreatic well differentiated NETs and a history of carcinoid syndrome were randomized to receive everolimus or placebo. While a trend towards improved progressive free survival was seen with the mTOR inhibitor, the results were not statistically significant, hence the agent is not approved for this indication. Phase III trials with a VEGF inhibitor have not been completed in carcinoid, although SWOG-0518 is ongoing (bevacizumab plus octreotide LAR vs. placebo plus octreotide LAR).

For patients with clinically significant progressive disease in the liver, liver directed therapy (e.g., arterial embolization, chemoembolization, radioembolization, or ablative therapy), may be considered although randomized trials are lacking (Nakakura, Venook et al. 2007). Accumulating data with peptide receptor radionuclide therapy (PRRT) suggest that this modality might hold promise for patients with advanced NETs (Bodei, Pepe et al. 2010).

4.2 Treatment of poorly differentiated (high grade) NETs of unknown primary

For patients with poorly differentiated (high grade) neuroendocrine carcinoma of unknown primary, chemotherapy with a small cell lung cancer regimen (i.e., platinum-based therapy, such as etoposide and cisplatin) should be considered (Nakakura, Venook et al. 2007;

Stoyianni, Pentheroudakis et al. 2011). A study of etoposide and cisplatin in patients with poorly differentiated NETs had an objective response rate of 41.5%, an 8.9 month median progression-free survival, and 15 month median overall survival (Mintry, Baudin et al. 1999). Other regimens include carboplatin- and irinotecan- based combinations, which are also small cell lung cancer regimens (Strosberg, Coppola et al. 2010). These tumors carry a poor prognosis.

4.3 Outcome of well differentiated (low and intermediate grade) unknown primary tumors

Patients with well differentiated neuroendocrine carcinoma of unknown primary may exhibit a relatively indolent course similar to those with advanced well differentiated NETs arising from the GI tract and BP tree (Stoyianni, Pentheroudakis et al. 2011). In a study by Kirshborn et al., patients with advanced midgut NETs (i.e., arising from the jejunum, ileum, and cecum) and those with neuroendocrine carcinoma of unknown primary shared similar serotonin levels as assessed by urine 24 hours hydroxyindoleacetic acid and serotonin levels, as well as by serum and platelet serotonin levels (Kirshbom, Kherani et al. 1998). Moreover, patients with advanced midgut NETs and neuroendocrine carcinoma of unknown primary shared similar 10-year survival rates (28% and 22%, respectively).

In a larger study, Yao et al. analyzed the outcomes of nearly 36,000 patients with NETs and found that primary site was probably the most useful predictor of outcome for patients with well differentiated NETs (Yao, Hassan et al. 2008). Patients with a liver primary and localized disease (i.e., disease confined to the liver) had a 5-year survival rate of 43%; this compared favorably with a 5-year survival rate of 54% for patients with a jejunum/ileum primary and distant disease. Not surprisingly, for patients with a liver primary and distant disease (i.e., widely metastatic disease), the prognosis was poor with a 0% survival rate at 10-years.

4.4 Outcome of poorly differentiated (high grade) NETs of unknown primary

Patients with poorly differentiated (high grade) neuroendocrine carcinoma of unknown primary clinically resemble those with aggressive small cell lung cancer (Nakakura, Venook et al. 2007; Stoyianni, Pentheroudakis et al. 2011). That is, their disease frequently responds to platinum-based therapy but inevitably becomes refractory. These patients have a poor prognosis with a median survival typically less than 1 year.

5. Conclusion

The diagnosis and management of patients with neuroendocrine carcinoma of unknown primary is challenging. Tumor grade directs treatment and is prognostic. Patients with well differentiated (low and intermediate grade) NETs may benefit from identification of the primary site because it may influence prognosis, but also because the available treatments we have are increasingly site-specific (e.g. octreotide for midgut tumors, and chemotherapy, everolimus and sunitinib for pancreatic NETs). In some settings, the type and timing of surgical intervention may also be dictated by the primary site. In contrast, patients with poorly differentiated (high grade) neuroendocrine carcinoma of unknown primary clinically resemble those with aggressive small cell lung cancer: Patients with advanced high grade tumors tend to experience an aggressive course (regardless of primary site). As such, they should be assessed for possible treatment with a small cell lung cancer regimen (i.e., platinum- or irinotecan-based chemotherapy regimens).

6. References

Agoff, S. N., L. W. Lamps, et al. (2000). Thyroid transcription factor-1 is expressed in extrapulmonary small cell carcinomas but not in other extrapulmonary neuroendocrine tumors. *Mod Pathol* 13(3): 238-242.

Bader, T. R., R. C. Semelka, et al. (2001). MRI of carcinoid tumors: spectrum of appearances in the gastrointestinal tract and liver. *J Magn Reson Imaging* 14(3): 261-269.

Bodei, L., G. Pepe, et al. (2010). Peptide receptor radionuclide therapy (PRRT) of neuroendocrine tumors with somatostatin analogues. *Eur Rev Med Pharmacol Sci* 14(4): 347-351.

Boudreaux, J. P., D. S. Klimstra, et al. (2010). The NANETS consensus guideline for the diagnosis and management of neuroendocrine tumors: well-differentiated neuroendocrine tumors of the Jejunum, Ileum, Appendix, and Cecum. *Pancreas* 39(6): 753-766.

Boudreaux, J. P., B. Putty, et al. (2005). Surgical treatment of advanced-stage carcinoid tumors: lessons learned. *Ann Surg* 241(6): 839-845; discussion 845-836.

Cai, Y. C., B. Banner, et al. (2001). Cytokeratin 7 and 20 and thyroid transcription factor 1 can help distinguish pulmonary from gastrointestinal carcinoid and pancreatic endocrine tumors. *Hum Pathol* 32(10): 1087-1093.

Chan, J. A. and M. H. Kulke (2011). New treatment options for patients with advanced neuroendocrine tumors. *Curr Treat Options Oncol* 12(2): 136-148.

Chen, H., J. M. Hardacre, et al. (1998). Isolated liver metastases from neuroendocrine tumors: does resection prolong survival? *J Am Coll Surg* 187(1): 88-92; discussion 92-83.

Chu, P., E. Wu, et al. (2000). Cytokeratin 7 and cytokeratin 20 expression in epithelial neoplasms: a survey of 435 cases. *Mod Pathol* 13(9): 962-972.

Cunningham, J. L., T. Diaz de Stahl, et al. (2011). Common pathogenetic mechanism involving human chromosome 18 in familial and sporadic ileal carcinoid tumors. *Genes Chromosomes Cancer* 50(2): 82-94.

Du, E. Z., P. Goldstraw, et al. (2004). TTF-1 expression is specific for lung primary in typical and atypical carcinoids: TTF-1-positive carcinoids are predominantly in peripheral location. *Hum Pathol* 35(7): 825-831.

Ekeblad, S., A. Sundin, et al. (2007). Temozolomide as monotherapy is effective in treatment of advanced malignant neuroendocrine tumors. *Clin Cancer Res* 13(10): 2986-2991.

Erlander, M. G., X. J. Ma, et al. (2011). Performance and clinical evaluation of the 92-gene real-time PCR assay for tumor classification. *J Mol Diagn* 13(5): 493-503.

Givi, B., S. J. Pommier, et al. (2006). Operative resection of primary carcinoid neoplasms in patients with liver metastases yields significantly better survival. *Surgery* 140(6): 891-897; discussion 897-898.

Haynes, C. M., A. R. Sangoi, et al. (2011). PAX8 is expressed in pancreatic well-differentiated neuroendocrine tumors and in extrapancreatic poorly differentiated neuroendocrine carcinomas in fine-needle aspiration biopsy specimens. *Cancer Cytopathol* 119(3): 193-201.

Hellman, P., T. Lundstrom, et al. (2002). Effect of surgery on the outcome of midgut carcinoid disease with lymph node and liver metastases. *World J Surg* 26(8): 991-997.

Jiao, Y., C. Shi, et al. (2011). DAXX/ATRX, MEN1, and mTOR pathway genes are frequently altered in pancreatic neuroendocrine tumors. *Science* 331(6021): 1199-1203.

Johanssen, S., M. Boivin, et al. (2006). The yield of wireless capsule endoscopy in the detection of neuroendocrine tumors in comparison with CT enteroclysis. *Gastrointest Endosc* 63(4): 660-665.

Khashab, M. A., E. Yong, et al. (2011). EUS is still superior to multidetector computerized tomography for detection of pancreatic neuroendocrine tumors. *Gastrointest Endosc* 73(4): 691-696.

Kirshbom, P. M., A. R. Kherani, et al. (1998). Carcinoids of unknown origin: comparative analysis with foregut, midgut, and hindgut carcinoids. *Surgery* 124(6): 1063-1070.

Klimstra, D. S., I. R. Modlin, et al. (2010). The pathologic classification of neuroendocrine tumors: a review of nomenclature, grading, and staging systems. *Pancreas* 39(6): 707-712.

Lin, X., R. S. Saad, et al. (2007). Diagnostic value of CDX-2 and TTF-1 expressions in separating metastatic neuroendocrine neoplasms of unknown origin. *Appl Immunohistochem Mol Morphol* 15(4): 407-414.

Makridis, C., K. Oberg, et al. (1990). Surgical treatment of mid-gut carcinoid tumors. *World J Surg* 14(3): 377-383; discussion 384-375.

Matoso, A., K. Singh, et al. (2009). Comparison of Thyroid Transcription Factor-1 Expression by 2 Monoclonal Antibodies in Pulmonary and Nonpulmonary Primary Tumors. *Appl Immunohistochem Mol Morphol.*

Modlin, I. M., M. D. Shapiro, et al. (2004). Siegfried Oberndorfer: origins and perspectives of carcinoid tumors. *Hum Pathol* 35(12): 1440-1451.

Nakakura, E. K., A. P. Venook, et al. (2007). Systemic and regional nonsurgical therapy--what is the optimal strategy for metastatic neuroendocrine cancer? *Surg Oncol Clin N Am* 16(3): 639-651, x.

Norton, J. A., D. L. Fraker, et al. (2006). Surgery increases survival in patients with gastrinoma. *Ann Surg* 244(3): 410-419.

Oberndorfer, S. (1907). Karzenoide tumoren des dunndarms. *FrankfZschr Pathol* 1: 426-432.

Oliveira, A. M., H. D. Tazelaar, et al. (2001). Thyroid transcription factor-1 distinguishes metastatic pulmonary from well-differentiated neuroendocrine tumors of other sites. *Am J Surg Pathol* 25(6): 815-819.

Picus, D., H. S. Glazer, et al. (1984). Computed tomography of abdominal carcinoid tumors. *AJR Am J Roentgenol* 143(3): 581-584.

Raymond, E., L. Dahan, et al. (2011). Sunitinib malate for the treatment of pancreatic neuroendocrine tumors. *N Engl J Med* 364(6): 501-513.

Rinke, A., H. H. Muller, et al. (2009). Placebo-controlled, double-blind, prospective, randomized study on the effect of octreotide LAR in the control of tumor growth in patients with metastatic neuroendocrine midgut tumors: a report from the PROMID Study Group. *J Clin Oncol* 27(28): 4656-4663.

Saqi, A., D. Alexis, et al. (2005). Usefulness of CDX2 and TTF-1 in differentiating gastrointestinal from pulmonary carcinoids. *Am J Clin Pathol* 123(3): 394-404.

Schmitt, A. M., F. Riniker, et al. (2008). Islet 1 (Isl1) expression is a reliable marker for pancreatic endocrine tumors and their metastases. *Am J Surg Pathol* 32(3): 420-425.

Srivastava, A. and J. L. Hornick (2009). Immunohistochemical staining for CDX-2, PDX-1, NESP-55, and TTF-1 can help distinguish gastrointestinal carcinoid tumors from pancreatic endocrine and pulmonary carcinoid tumors. *Am J Surg Pathol* 33(4): 626-632.

Stoyianni, A., G. Pentheroudakis, et al. (2011). Neuroendocrine carcinoma of unknown primary: a systematic review of the literature and a comparative study with other neuroendocrine tumors. *Cancer Treat Rev* 37(5): 358-365.

Strosberg, J. R., A. Cheema, et al. (2011). A review of systemic and liver-directed therapies for metastatic neuroendocrine tumors of the gastroenteropancreatic tract. *Cancer Control* 18(2): 127-137.

Strosberg, J. R., D. Coppola, et al. (2010). The NANETS consensus guidelines for the diagnosis and management of poorly differentiated (high-grade) extrapulmonary neuroendocrine carcinomas. *Pancreas* 39(6): 799-800.

Strosberg, J. R., R. L. Fine, et al. (2011). First-line chemotherapy with capecitabine and temozolomide in patients with metastatic pancreatic endocrine carcinomas. *Cancer* 117(2): 268-275.

Sugimoto, E., L. E. Lorelius, et al. (1995). Midgut carcinoid tumours. CT appearance. *Acta Radiol* 36(4): 367-371.

van Tuyl, S. A., E. J. Kuipers, et al. (2004). Video capsule endoscopy: procedure, indications and diagnostic yield. *Neth J Med* 62(7): 225-228.

Wang, S. C., J. R. Parekh, et al. (2010). Identification of unknown primary tumors in patients with neuroendocrine liver metastases. *Arch Surg* 145(3): 276-280.

Wang, Y. C., E. Gallego-Arteche, et al. (2009). Homeodomain transcription factor NKX2.2 functions in immature cells to control enteroendocrine differentiation and is expressed in gastrointestinal neuroendocrine tumors. *Endocr Relat Cancer* 16(1): 267-279.

Wang, Y. C., G. Iezza, et al. (2010). Lack of NKX2.2 expression in bronchopulmonary typical carcinoid tumors: implications for patients with neuroendocrine tumor metastases and unknown primary site. *J Surg Res* 163(1): 47-51.

Welin, S., H. Sorbye, et al. (2011). Clinical effect of temozolomide-based chemotherapy in poorly differentiated endocrine carcinoma after progression on first-line chemotherapy. *Cancer.*

Yao, J. C., M. Hassan, et al. (2008). One hundred years after "carcinoid": epidemiology of and prognostic factors for neuroendocrine tumors in 35,825 cases in the United States. *J Clin Oncol* 26(18): 3063-3072.

Yao, J. C., M. H. Shah, et al. (2011). Everolimus for advanced pancreatic neuroendocrine tumors. *N Engl J Med* 364(6): 514-523.

5

Gastrointestinal Neuroendocrine Tumors

Ozcan Yildiz and Suheyla Serdengecti
Istanbul University/Cerrahpasa Medical Faculty,Department of Internal Medicine, Division of Medical Oncology Istanbul, Turkey

1. Introduction

Gastrointestinal carcinoid tumors date back to 1888 when Otto Lubarsch found multiple tumors in the distal ileum of two patients at autopsy (Lubarsch, 1888). The German pathologist Siegfried Oberndorfer was the first who used the term "Karzinoide Tumoren", the English translation of which is "carcinoid tumor". He coined this term because these tumors behaved less aggressively than true carcinomas (Oberndorfer, 1907). Oberndorfer contributed to the Department of Pathology of Istanbul University where he remained full professor and director until his death in 1944 (Dogan & Hot, 2010; Klöppel et al., 2007). In 1914, Gosset and Masson first mentioned neuroendocrine features of carcinoid tumors. In 1954, Thorson and co-workers described the term "carcinoid syndrome" after they found that the tumors contained serotonin and patients with small intestinal carcinoid tumor and liver metastases presented with the characteristic symptoms of diarrhea, flushing, asthma, and right heart failure (Thorson et al., 1954). It was soon recognized as a distinct entity after they were reported in several organs belonging to bronchopulmonary system and gastrointestinal tract (Yalcin, 2006). Although better named as "neuroendocrine tumors" after the WHO meeting in 2000, these tumors have been traditionally called "carcinoids" especially at some specific locations such as the gastrointestinal tract. Therefore, the terms "carcinoid tumor" and "neuroendocrine tumor" are used interchangeably throughout the text.

2. Epidemiology

Although it might not reflect the true incidence due to their indolent nature, the overall incidence of carcinoid tumors in the United.States has been estimated to be 1 to 2 cases per 100,000 people (Godwin, 1975; Modlin & Sandor, 1997). Yao and co-workers reviewed 35,825 neuroendocrine tumors (NETs) compiled from 1973 to 2004 (Yao et al., 2008). According to this review, 41% was foregut NETs, 26% midgut NETs, and 19% hindgut NETs. In the remaining 13%, the primary tumor site was unknown or could not be classified. These figures were similar to our institution's patient cohort (Yildiz et al., 2009). In Sweden, combined with the autopsy series the incidence has been calculated to be 8.4 cases per 100,000 people. Based on the data from the End Results Group (1950-1969) and the Third National Cancer Survey (1969-1971) the most common site of carcinoid tumors was appendix followed by the rectum, ileum, lung and bronchi, and stomach (Godwin, 1975). Pancreatic endocrine tumors are relatively less frequent and account for 2% of malignant tumors of the gastrointestinal tract. Recent data obtained from the National Cancer Institute Surveillance, Epidemiology, and End Results program (1973 to 1997) showed that, of the 11,427 cases analyzed, the overall incidence rates for carcinoid tumors have increased significantly over the past 25 years, although rates for some sites have decreased (e.g., appendix). The gastrointestinal tract accounted for 54.5% of the tumors. Within the gastrointestinal tract, the small intestine was the most common site (44.7%), followed by the rectum (19.6%), appendix (16.7%), colon (10.6%), and stomach (7.2%). The average age was 60.9 years, and 54.2% were female. The 5-year survival rates for the most common gastrointestinal sites were 75.1% for stomach, 76.1% for small intestine, 76.3% for appendix, and 87.5% for rectum (Maggard et al., 2004).

3. Pathology and classification

Carcinoid tumors are thought to arise primarily from the neuroendocrine cells of the lung and the gastrointestinal tract. In the past, these cells were called "Kulchitsky cells" or "enterochromaffin cells" due to the affinity for soluble silver salts, hence the term argentaffinomas. Although not prognostically useful, historically, carcinoid tumors have been classified according to their embryologic derivation within the primitive gut (Williams & Sandler, 1963): Foregut, midgut, and hindgut carcinoids. Foregut carcinoids include intrathoracic (thymic and bronchial), gastric, esophageal, upper duodenal, and pancreatic carcinoids. They usually produce low levels of serotonin, 5-hydroxytryptophan (5-HTP), histamine, or adrenocorticotropic hormone. Midgut carcinoids include carcinoids of distal duodenum, jejunum, ileum, appendix, proximal colon, liver, ovary, or testes. These tumors have the propensity of producing serotonin at high levels. Finally, hindgut carcinoids include carcinoids of distal colon and rectum. They less likely produce serotonin but may produce somatostatin, peptide YY, 5-HTP, or other hormones (Table 1).

Useful immunohistochemical markers in modern pathology include neuron-specific enolase (NSE), synapthophysin and chromogranin A (CgA) which is also a secretory product of the carcinoid cells used to monitor disease activity (Table 2). On gross examination, carcinoid tumors are small yellow nodules located submucosally. When they invade the serosa, an intense desmoplastic reaction occurs that may lead to intestinal kinking and obstruction.

The WHO 1980 classification had taken into account the histologic features apart from the site of origin (Bosman et al., 2010; table 3). According to this revised system, well-differentiated neuroendocrine tumors are typical tumors that show characteristic growth pattern and benign behavior. They are indolent tumors, confined to mucosa or submucosa, and less than 1 to 2 cm in diameter.

In the WHO 2000 classification, features such as differentiation and proliferation were retained, but location, tumor size, tumor extent, and angioinvasion were transferred into the TNM (Tumor, Node, Metastasis) staging classification. The WHO 2010 classification states that all GEP-NETs are potentially malignant, but differ in their ability of metastasis (Rindi et al., 2010). Well-differentiated NETs are classified together as neuroendocrine tumors (NETs) G1 or G2. NET G1 is analogous with carcinoid. The term neuroendocrine carcinoma (NEC), unlike NET, refers to all poorly differentiated NETs. NEC is further subdivided into a small-cell and a large-cell variant. In respect of proliferation, all NECs are actively proliferating G3 tumors. Mixed adenoneuroendocrine carcinomas (MANEC) and hyperplastic and preneoplastic lesions are special groups. This classification is complemented by GEP-NET-specific TNM classifications and a grading system, which improves prognostic and treatment stratification (Schott et al., 2011).

Secretory products of carcinoid tumors	**Frequency (%)**
Amines	
5-Hydroxytrypta mine	-
5-Hydroxyindoleacetic acid	88
5-Hydroxytryptophan	-
5-Hydroxyindoleacetaldehyde	-
Histamine	-
Dopamine	-
Tachykinins	-
Kallikrein	-
Substance P	32
Neuropeptide K	66
Peptides	
Pancreatic polypeptide	43
Chromogranins	100
Neurotensin	41
Human chorionic gonadotrophin-alpha	28
Human chorionic gonadotropin-beta	12
Motilin	14
Pancreastatin	-
Other	
Prostaglandins	-

(O'Dorisio, 2011; Vinik et al., 2008; Norheim et al., 1987; Feldmann & O'Dorisio 1986; Eriksson et al., 1990)

Table 1. Secretory products and known frequency of carcinoid tumors

Foregut	**Midgut**	**Hindgut**
Argyrophilic	*Argentaffin-positive*	*Argyrophilic*
CgA-positive	CgA-positive	CgA-positive
NSE-positive	NSE-positive	NSE-positive
Synaptophysin-positive	Synaptophysin-positive	Synaptophysin-positive
		SVP-2-positive

CgA: Chromogranin A; SVP-2: Seminal vesicle protein-2; NSE: neuron specific enolase

Table 2. Immunestaining of carcinoid tumors regarding their embryonic origin

Well-differentiated endocrine tumors may exhibit uncertain behavior. They may be angioinvasive. They may also produce serotonin and enteroglucagon. Another subset is well-differentiated endocrine carcinomas once termed "atypical" or "anaplastic". They are subdivided into low-grade and high-grade malignant carcinoids. Low-grade malignant carcinoids are deeply invasive (muscularis propria or beyond) and serotonin-producing when metastatic disease develops. High-grade malignant carcinoids, on the other hand, are small to intermediate carcinomas. Appendiceal and rectal carcinoids are rarely malignant, whereas ileal, type III gastric, and colonic ones are frequently malignant. Size is also a predictor of the malignant potential of the carcinoid tumor. More than 66% of carcinoids greater than 2 cm exhibit distant spread when first diagnosed (Capella et al., 1995).

	WHO 1980		WHO 2000		WHO 2010
I.	Carcinoid	1.	Well-differentiated differentiated endocrine tumor (WDET)	1.	Neuroendocrine tumor G1 (Carcinoid)
		2.	Well-differentiated endocrine carcinoma (WDEC)	2.	NET G2
		3.	Poorly differentiated (small-cell) endocrine carcinoma (PDEC)	3.	Small or large-cell neuroendocrine carcinoma G3 (NEC)
II. III.	Mucocarcinoid Mixed carcinoid-adenocarcinoma	4.	Mixed endocrine-exocrine carcinoma (MEEC)	5.	Mixed adenoneuroendocrine carcinoma
IV.	Pseudotumorous lesion	6.	Tumor-like lesions (TLL)	7.	Hyperplastic and preneoplastic lesion

Table 3. Comparison of the WHO classifications of gastroenteropancreatic neuroendocrine tumors. Bosman FT, et al., WHO classification of tumors of the digestive system. Lyon, France: IARC Press; 2010.

4. Clinical chemistry

Clinically functioning carcinoid tumors produce typical syndromes according to the specific circulating peptide. One of the best-characterized of these peptides is serotonin (5-HT). It is synthesized from 5-hydroxytryptophan (5-HTP) and metabolized to 5-hydroxyindoleacetic acid (5-HIAA) which is excreted in the urine. Measurement of 5-HIAA in the urine is an important tumor marker in the carcinoid syndrome, especially in midgut carcinoids. Recently, measurements of serotonin in platelets have been recommended for the detection of carcinoid tumors that secrete only small amounts of serotonin and/or its precursor 5-hydroxytryptophan (Kema et al., 2000). Tumors originating from foregut carcinoids (lung, pancreas, and stomach) may have relatively low levels of 5-HTP decarboxylase. 5-HTP, 5-HT, and 5-HIAA are excreted in the urine.

5. Clinical features of individual carcinoids

5.1 Foregut carcinoids

For the sake of completeness we will discuss thymic and pulmonary carcinoids in the following sections.

5.1.1 Thymic carcinoids

Thymic carcinoids are rare and may be part of multiple endocrine neoplasia type 1 (MEN1). The tumor is usually non-functioning and occurs as an anterior mediastinal mass. The mass may be partly calcified and may cause superior vena cava obstruction. Extension into the pleura, pericardium, great vessels, or regional lymph nodes is commonly seen. Functioning thymic carcinoids usually secrete adrenocorticotrophic hormone (ACTH), which may lead to Cushing's syndrome. In these cases bilateral adrenal hyperplasia may also be seen. Other hormones include corticotrophin-releasing hormone, growth hormone-releasing hormone (GHRH) and 5-HT. Carcinoid syndrome has been described with a multidirectional carcinoma of the thymus with neuroendocrine and sarcomatous components. (Paties et al., 1991)

5.1.2 Pulmonary carcinoids

Pulmonary carcinoid tumors comprise about 2% of primary lung tumors. They are believed to arise from neuroendocrine Kulchitsky's cells of the proximal bronchial mucosa, and bronchopulmonary tract is the second common site of carcinoid tumors after the gastrointestinal system. They have been classified into three groups, according to their malignant potential: Benign or classical bronchial carcinoid, low-grade malignant or atypical carcinoid, and high-grade malignant or poorly differentiated carcinoma of the large cell or small cell type.

Neuroendocrine tumors of the lung can also be divided into 5 groups: Tumorlet, diffuse idiopathic pulmonary neuroendocrine cell hyperplasia (DIPNECH) (Nassar et al., 2011), carcinoid tumor, atypical carcinoid tumor, and small cell carcinoma of the lung. Typical carcinoids of the lung present in the fifth decade of life and are more common in females. These tumors are not related to smoking. Neuroendocrine manifestations are relatively uncommon. Common symptoms are cough, hemoptysis, wheezing, and chest pain (Table 4). Recurrent pneumonia can occur due to obstructing lesions. Cushing's syndrome and acromegaly may be seen due to the secretion of ACTH and GHRH, respectively. The prognosis is excellent for classical bronchial carcinoids. Diagnostic tools for pulmonary carcinoids are generally non-specific. Bronchoscopic biopsy should be used to obtain diagnostic tissue, despite the feared complication of hemorrhage.

Carcinoid tumors	Clinical features
Foregut	
Bronchial carcinoids	Cough, hemoptysis, wheezing, chest pain, pneumonia
Gastric carcinoids	Usually found incidentally
Midgut	
Small intestinal carcinoids	Bowel obstruction
Appendiceal carcinoids	Nonspecific abdominal pain, carcinoid syndrome Usually found incidentally
Hindgut	
Rectal carcinoids	Bleeding, pain, constipation, carcinoid syndrome

Table 4. Clinical features of neuroendocrine tumors

Treatment should not be radical unless there is lymph node metastasis. Options include lobectomy, segmentectomy, and bronchotomy with tumor enucleation. Curative or palliative metastasectomies are worth trying since they grow slowly. Carcinoid crisis should be prevented with octreotide administration preoperatively. When chemotherapy is indicated in some patients, 5-fluorouracil and streptozotosin or cisplatin and etoposide are most commonly used regimens. Other drugs used in metastatic pulmonary carcinoids are octreotide, 131I-MIBG, and interferon alpha. Stage-by-stage, the outcome is worse for patients with atypical carcinoids than for those with typical carcinoids (Kaplan et al., 2003).

5.1.3 Gastric carcinoids

Gastric carcinoids are rare neoplasms of the stomach comprising less than 1% of gastric tumors and 8.7% of all gastrointestinal neuroendocrine tumors (Godwin, 1975; Modlin et al., 1997) (Table 4). The incidence is reported to be 1.2 and 1.8/1,000,000 persons/year in white males and females, respectively. Three types have been described: Those associated with chronic atrophic gastritis type A (CAG-A or type I), those associated with Zollinger-Ellison syndrome (type II), and sporadic gastric carcinoid tumors (type III). The first 2 groups of carcinoids are associated with hypergastrinemia. CAG-A associated carcinoids are the most common type (70-80% of cases). The typical patient is a woman in her sixties with pernicious anemia, hypochlorhydria, and hypergastrinemia. High levels of gastrin may mediate the hyperplasia of enterochromaffin-like (ECL) cells in the gastric mucosa and ultimately, carcinoid tumors may develop. They are small indolent, non-functioning tumors and located multifocally in the body or fundus, which are diagnosed incidentally (Rindi et al., 1993; Gough et al., 1994; Moses et al., 1986). Tumors less than 1 cm have been successfully resected and followed endoscopically (Ahlman et al., 1994; Sjoblom et al., 1993). Gastric carcinoids associated with the Zollinger-Ellison syndrome (ZES) almost always occur in patients with multiple endocrine neoplasia type 1 (MEN1 or Wermer's syndrome) suggesting a genetic predisposition. Five percent of gastric carcinoids are of type II. The treatment and prognosis are similar to those of CAG-A associated carcinoids. Within this group, there is also a non-MEN1 associated sporadic ZES which rarely leads to gastric carcinoid tumor development. Interestingly, 99% of them had ECL hyperplasia and abnormal alpha-human chorionic gonadotropin (a-hCG) staining. Sporadic gastric carcinoids (type III), in contrast, are not associated with hypergastrinemia and follow an aggressive clinical course. In addition to being solitary, they are usually more than 1 cm in size and often metastatic at the time of diagnosis. When feasible, radical gastrectomy is the treatment of choice.

5.2 Midgut carcinoids

5.2.1 Small intestinal carcinoids

Small bowel is not only the most frequent site of carcinoid tumors (including metastatic carcinoids), but also carcinoids are the commonest primary malignant tumor of the distal small intestine. Their frequency has recently surpassed adenocarcinoma (44% versus 33%) (Bilimoria et al., 2009). More than one third of the small bowel tumors are diagnosed as carcinoids and of all gastrointestinal carcinoids; 42% arise in the small bowel of which the ileum represents the most common localization followed by the duodenum and the jejunum. The annual incidence rate is 0,28 per 100,000. Patients usually present in 6th or 7th decade of life with mechanical obstruction or vague abdominal pain, sometimes for several years before the diagnosis perhaps due to their submucosal location. These tumors are thought to originate from serotonin-producing intraepithelial endocrine cells and they tend to have high serotonin content. They are multicentric and the most frequent location is the distal ileum. Lymph node and liver metastasis are common but carcinoid syndrome is seen only in 5 to 7% of the patients (Burke et al., 1997; Bilimoria et al., 2009). Metastases tend to occur in liver, bone and lung. Unlike appendiceal carcinoids, smaller tumors have also been found to have metastasized. Nevertheless, tumors measuring 2 cm in diameter have almost always been proved to have distant spreading.

Based on patients, registered in the Swedish Cancer Registry, with small intestinal carcinoids diagnosed from 1960 to 2000 in the duodenum (n= 89) and jejunum/ileum (n=2437), the overall 5-, 10-, and 15 year survivals were, respectively, 60, 46, and 28% for duodenal tumors and 56, 36, and 23% for jejunal/ileal tumors (Zar et al., 2004).

5.2.2 Appendiceal carcinoids

Carcinoid tumors are the most common cancers of the appendix (Moertel et al., 1968) originating from subepithelial endocrine cells (Lundqvist & Wilander, 1986; Shaw, 1990). They are detected most commonly after appendectomy performed for other reasons and they are found in 0.3-0.9% of patients undergoing appendectomy (Goede et al., 2003). Median age is 4th or 5th decade of life (Modlin & Sandor, 1997). This age range is partly explained by higher appendectomy rate in young adults. Less than 10% of appendiceal carcinoids cause symptoms due to the distal localization of the tumor (Moertel et al., 1987). However, they become symptomatic earlier than the carcinoids of other sites. This may also explain the relatively less frequent metastasis of appendiceal carcinoids regarding tumor size. On the other hand, the size of the tumor is the best predictor of outcome according to the Mayo Clinic series. The critical size has been found to be 2 cm. Therefore, right hemicolectomy is the treatment of choice for those tumors that are more than 2 cm in size as well as those located at the base of the appendix regardless of their size. Local desmoplasia is another indication of right hemicolectomy. Otherwise simple appendectomy suffices as there is no evidence of recurrence after a median follow-up of more than 25 years in the appropriate age group (Moertel et al., 1987).

5.3 Hindgut carcinoids

5.3.1 Colonic carcinoids

Less than 1% of colon cancers are carcinoids (Modlin IM, 1997). The usual presentation of colonic carcinoids in patients is bleeding, pain and obstruction (Table 3). In a study of 72 patients, the more common symptoms were pain, anorexia and weight loss (Rosenberg JM, 1985). Patients were usually at their 7th decade of life. The most common location was cecum. Midgut colonic carcinoids, namely proximal colonic ones, are believed to arise from serotonin-secreting epithelial endocrine cells, behave more aggressively and symptomatic tumors need to be approached radically. Fulguration should be avoided in colonic carcinoids due to a risk of perforation. As for prognosis, 5-year survival rate is 70% in patients with local disease; 44% and 20% in patients with regional metastases and distant spread, respectively.

5.3.2 Rectal carcinoids

Rectal carcinoids constitute 1 to 2% of all rectal cancers and are the most common hindgut carcinoid. They occur most commonly in the 6th decade of life (Modlin & Sandor, 1997). Recent series have shown that they are relatively common (Matsui et al., 1993; Jemore et al., 1992). In one series between 1992 and 1999, they accounted for 27% of all gastrointestinal carcinoid tumors (Modlin et al., 2003). Unlike other carcinoids, they do not usually produce serotonin and therefore do not cause carcinoid syndrome despite extensive metastases. Symptomatic patients have rectal bleeding, pain, and constipation (Table 4) (Harpole et al., 1992; Smith, 1969). They are submucosally located and almost always diagnosed with endoscopic biopsies. Size is the major factor for metastasis. Tumors less than 1 cm in diameter has never been shown to have metastasized during a follow up of up to 25 years according to the Mayo Clinic experience. However, tumors more than 2 cm, which make up about 5%, behave aggressively. For patients with tumors between 1 cm and 2 cm, an individualized approach is appropriate considering age and comorbid conditions.

6. Carcinoid syndrome

The clinical presentation of the carcinoid tumors varies depending on localization, hormone production, and extent of disease. Midgut carcinoids often present with bowel obstruction or abdominal pain. Patients with rectal carcinoids often seek medical attention with bleeding. Lung carcinoids are found incidentally or they may secrete ACTH or CRH to present with Cushing's syndrome. Growth hormone-releasing hormone secreted by foregut carcinoids may cause acromegaly. Duodenal carcinoids may cause somatostatinoma syndrome. However, the most characteristic clinical feature of carcinoid tumors is carcinoid syndrome.

Carcinoid syndrome, which is almost always seen when the tumor has metastasized to the liver, is the third most common mode of presentation of carcinoid tumors after bowel obstruction and abdominal pain. A small proportion of midgut carcinoids without liver metastasis can still present with carcinoid syndrome suggesting direct liberation of the causative agents into the systemic circulation. Flushing and diarrhea are the most common components of carcinoid syndrome, which are seen up to 89% of the patients during their course of the disease. Flushing is characterized by a sudden onset, deep red or violaceous erythema of the upper body often associated with a feeling of warmth. It is the prominent symptom in midgut carcinoids, which is thought to be due to catecholamine induced kallikrein release. In bronchial carcinoids, the flushing is usually prolonged sometimes hours or days giving rise to permanent dilatation of facial veins and telangiectasia. Gastric carcinoids may cause a characteristic flush that is reddish in color and pachy in distribution reminiscent of an urticarial reaction, which may be inhibited by histamine antagonists (Adamson et al., 1969). Other manifestations include asthma, edema, right heart vulvular lesions, the most common of which is tricuspid regurgitation, a loud sound of the pulmonic component of the 2nd heart sound, pellegra-like skin lesions, peptic ulcer, and arthralgia. Malignant carcinoid syndrome denotes patients with these manifestations combined with liver metastasis and elevated urinary 5-HIAA levels. Some patients may display only a few of the above signs. Usually, a full-blown carcinoid syndrome is seen in patients with extensive hepatic metastases. Some patients may have hepatic metastases with minimal symptoms and they generally look well. Ovarian and bronchial carcinoids may cause carcinoid syndrome without documented liver metastasis. While patients with small intestinal and proximal colonic carcinoids produce carcinoid syndrome most commonly, it is less commonly seen in bronchial carcinoids and does not occur in rectal carcinoids (Harpole et al., 1992; Smith, 1969; Caldarola et al., 1964). Due to the vagueness of the symptoms or no symptoms at all, diagnosis is delayed approximately 2 to 3 years (Norheim et al., 1987).

7. Diagnosis

The diagnosis of a carcinoid tumor depends on the symptomatology of carcinoid syndrome or the presence of other symptoms such as abdominal discomfort. Nevertheless, 60% of the patients with gastrointestinal carcinoids found at surgery were asymptomatic in one study (Thompson et al., 1985). The histopathologic diagnosis is made using immunohistochemical techniques, namely antibodies directed against chromogranin A (CgA), synaptophysin, and NSE. In patients with carcinoid syndrome the diagnosis can be made measuring urinary 5-HIAA levels. Levels of 15 to 60 mg/24 hours are compatible with midgut carcinoid tumors with 60 to 73% of sensitivity and 100% specificity. The most sensitive marker is plasma CgA, albeit not specific, since other neuroendocrine tumors can secrete this substance. Foregut carcinoids, on the other hand, may produce an atypical carcinoid syndrome with minimally elevated or normal urinary 5-HIAA level since they lack the enzyme L-amino-acid decarboxylase. The diagnosis of these tumors rely upon measurement of urinary metabolites of tryptophan such as 5-HTP or 5-HT. Patients should abstain from bananas, avocado, pineapple, walnuts, chocolate, and coffee; and avoid drugs such as chlorpromazine (Bertino & Cole, 1956) salicylates, and L-dopa at least 24 hours before the sample is presented to the lab (DeVita et al., 2011).

8. Localization

After the diagnosis has been made localization should be determined for the optimal management of the carcinoid tumor. Bronchial carcinoids are located in the airways of the central or middle third of the lung in 80% of cases. Chest x-ray, computed tomography (CT) or bronchoscopy is used to detect these tumors (Nessi et al., 1991). In plain radiography, they appear as a well-demarcated round or ovoid mass, often notched. Small tumors, which are often the case, are best detected by CT scanning. The mass may be visible within the bronchial lumina with an extraluminal component. In peripheral lesions, the mass is typically round or ovoid with a smooth or lobulated border. MRI is reserved for cases in which pulmonary carcinoid is suspected but cannot be visualized on CT.

As midgut carcinoids are small tumors, they are sometimes detected by angiography or somatostatin-receptor scintigraphy (SRS) if not detected by barium enema, CT or MRI. Secondary features such as liver metastases and bowel obstruction are more often visualized than the primary tumor. Liver metastasis can be visualized by CT or MRI. Positron emission tomography (PET) using 11C-5-HTP is another localization modality with a high sensitivity (Orlefors et al., 1998; Sundin et al., 2004). Echocardiography should be performed in all patients with carcinoid syndrome to detect signs of carcinoid heart disease which is associated with poor survival.

Hindgut carcinoids are usually localized at endoscopy. They appear as solitary yellowish submucosal lesions. Endoscopic ultrasound may demonstrate invasion of the full rectal wall (stage T3) or adjacent structures (T4).

In recent years, SRS or octreoscan and iodinated meta-iodobenzylguanidine (123I-MIBG) have been introduced to localize and stage the tumor. Five somatostatin receptors are currently recognized bound to varying degrees by the analogues 111In-octreotide, 111In-lanreotide, and P829, a new technetium-99m (99mTc) analogue (Menda & Khan, 2002). Octreotide receptor imaging is most useful for the prediction of the success of octreotide therapy. If the scan is positive, then therapy will most likely be beneficial. It is also used peroperatively for perioperative tumor detection. Imaging with 123I-MIBG can also be performed for the prediction of therapy success with 131I-MIBG. The frequency of positive imaging in carcinoid tumors is 50-75% for 123I-MIBG and 67-96% for 111ln-octreotide. 123I-MIBG scintigraphy, which is more widely available, appears to be more sensitive for sympatho-adrenomedullary tumors such as pheochromocytomas and paragangliomas, whereas 111ln-octreotide detects more tumors in all other neuroendocrine neoplasms.

9. Management of carcinoid tumors

Tumor reduction and symptomatic control are the mainstays of treatment of carcinoid tumors. When the tumor is localized, surgical resection the extent of which is determined primarily by the tumor size, is the treatment of choice. Symptomatic control includes lifestyle changes, dietary supplementation, and medical treatments directed to specific symptoms of carcinoid syndrome. Benign cases can respond to avoiding physical and emotional stress, alcohol, spicy food, and certain drugs. Supplemental niacin is recommended in patients whose symptoms are due to serotonin excess to prevent pellegra. Heart failure due to carcinoid heart disease requires drugs such as angiotensin-converting enzyme (ACE) inhibitors and diuretics. Diarrhea may respond to loperamide or diphenoxylate. Side effects of these drugs are the main limiting factor in controlling carcinoid syndrome. Therefore, more specific drugs have been developed, one of which is octreotide, a somatostatin analogue.

9.1 Surgical palliation

Patients suspected with intestinal obstruction must be relieved of their obstruction even if they have extensive liver metastases. Liver metastases can be resected without jeopardizing survival in select patients (Que et al., 1995; McEntee et al., 1990; & Dousset, 1996). Liver resection has been associated with improved 5 year survival rates in several series and is recommended in appropriate patients to attempt cure or to debulk metastatic disease (Sutton et al., 2003). Embolization of the hepatic artery is another option for liver disease. Liver transplantation for highly selected patients offers a five-year survival rate of 69% according to a French study (Le Treut et al., 1997). Mesenteric ischemia should promptly be recognized and the affected bowel segment resected.

9.2 Somatostatin analogues

Somatostatin analogues interact with cellular and transmembrane somatostatin receptors coupled with G proteins. Five subtypes have been defined. Subtypes 2, 3 and 5 are most important and somatostatin analogues exert their action primarily by binding to subtype 2 (Kubota et al., 1994). Activation results in inhibition of growth factor production and release as well as antiproliferative effects (Scarpignato & Pelosini, 2001; Buscail et al., 1995; Cordelier et al., 1997 & Cattaneo et al., 1996). Receptor subtype 3 mediates phosphotyrosine phosphatase dependent apoptosis during high dose therapy (3mg daily octreotide or 12 mg daily lanreotide) (Imam et al., 1997). Octreotide is the most widely available drug followed by lanreotide and vapreotide. Subcutaneous administration of these drugs can control the symptoms in most of the patients. The recommended dose of immediate release form of octreotide is 100 mcg 2 or 3 times a day. The dose should be titrated upwards according to the symptoms sometimes up to 3000 mcg a day in 3 to 7 days. Tolerance is a common caveat in long-term use. Long-acting, slow-release formulation of octreotide with 20 and 30 mg of doses (up to 60 mg) every month (every 2 weeks for lanreotide) has enabled patients to enjoy a more comfortable life in terms of controlling symptoms and reducing the number of injections. The immediate release formulation and the long-acting form should overlap at least 2 weeks to achieve maximal symptom control. Patients with breakthrough symptoms may benefit from subcutaneous administration of the immediate release formulation. Treatment should be continued life-long or until troublesome side effects develop. Somatostatin analogues improve symptoms in 88% of patients and in 72%, urinary 5-HIAA excretion decreases (Kvols et al., 1986).

9.3 Chemotherapy

Metastatic carcinoid tumors are indolent tumors and response to chemotherapeutics is generally poor. Classical midgut carcinoids do not show any response to chemotherapy. Since foregut carcinoids are more malignant than others, cytotoxic therapy can be attempted. Combinations include streptozotocin plus 5-fluorouracil, doxorubicin, cisplatin plus etoposide, and dacarbazine plus 5-fluorouracil (Moertel et al., 1991; Di Bartolomeo et al., 1995 & Bajetta et al., 1998). Somatostatin analogues can be combined with the above regimens. A recent study showed that chemotherapy naïve patients with metastatic pancreatic endocrine carcinomas had an exceptionally high and durable response rate with the combination of temezolamide and capecitabine (Strosberg et al., 2011).

9.4 Immunotherapy

Oberg and his coworkers have reported a study form Sweden that 42% of patients with carcinoid syndrome had a reduction of their urinary 5-HIAA levels when treated with low dose human leukocyte interferon and recombinant leukocyte interferon-a (Oberg et al., 1986), but there was only 11% tumor regression rate. Mayo Clinic tried higher doses of interferon (Moertel et al., 1991) and objective tumor regression was 20% but it was not durable. Toxicity was the major drawback. Oberg has suggested the dose of interferon be titrated according to the patient's neutrophil count.

9.5 Angiogenesis inhibitors

As neuroendocrine tumors are highly vascular tumors bevacizumab, a monoclonal antibody targeting vascular endothelial growth factor (VEGF), was tested in advanced neuroendocrine tumors. This phase II study resulted in objective responses, reduction of tumor blood flow, and longer PFS in patients with carcinoid than PEG interferon treatment (Yao, 2008). Sunitinib, another molecule inhibiting VEGF receptors, is approved by FDA for the treatment of advanced or unresectable progressive well-differentiated pancreatic neuroendocrine tumors based on the phase III study stating that it improves progression-free survival, overall survival, and the objective response rate of these tumors as compared with placebo (Raymond et al., 2011).

9.6 Mammalian target of rapamycin (mTOR) inhibitors

Everolimus inhibits mTOR, an intracellular serine/threonine kinase that regulates multiple signaling pahways. It showed activity in advanced or unresectable low-grade or intermediate-grade pancreatic neuroendocrine tumors (Yao et al., 2011) and approved by FDA for the treatment of advanced, unresctable, or locally advanced pancreatic neuroendocrine tumors.

9.7 Radiation therapy

External irradiation has been used for the palliation of bone and brain metastases (Schupak & Wallner, 1991 & Kimmig, 1994). Radiolabeled MIBG has been the most widely studied agent. It showed a 30% response rate with 125I-MIBG or 131I-MIBG (Hoefnagel et al., 1987 & Taal et al., 1996). In one study, investigators performed a retrospective review of 98 patients with metastatic carcinoid who were treated at their institution with 131I-MIBG over a 15-year period. The median survival after treatment was 2.3 years. Patients who experienced a symptomatic response had improved survival. For the 56 patients who had 5-HIAA levels monitored, the mean urine 5-HIAA levels decreased significantly after 131I-MIBG treatment. Authors concluded that 131I-MIBG treatment could be recommended in select patients with metastatic carcinoid who progress despite optimal medical management. Improved survival was predicted best by symptomatic response to 131I-MIBG treatment, but not by hormone or radiographic response (Safford et al., 2004). 111In-octreotide is a somatostatin analogue-based tumor-targeted radioactive agent. It is most often used when imaging with 123I-MIBG fails to detect any tumor. When 111In-octreotide is avidly concentrated within the tumors, then radionuclide labeled octreotide can be administered. Studies with 90Y-labeled octreotide have shown that 83% of patients with carcinoid syndrome had a significant reduction in symptoms (Waldherr et al., 2001).

9.8 Carcinoid heart disease

In the pre-somatostatin era carcinoid heart disease used to occur in two thirds of patients with the carcinoid syndrome (Lundin et al., 1988). However, in the post-somatostatin era its incidence has dropped dramatically to 5% (Anthony et al., 2011). Right heart is affected most commonly. Tricuspid regurgitation, tricuspid stenosis, pulmonary regurgitation, and pulmonary stenosis may all occur. It is thought that these lesions are due to the secreted factors by the carcinoid cells of the liver metastases into the hepatic vein. Serotonin is blamed to be responsible for the cardiac lesions in carcinoid syndrome. However, its role in the development of cardiac lesions is poorly understood. Left heart is less often affected due to inactivation of serotonin by lung metabolism. Valvular replacement in patients with symptomatic heart disease proved unsuccessful due to the high perioperative mortality (Robiolio et al., 1995 & Connolly et al., 1995).

10. Prognosis

Carcinoid syndrome represents an advanced disease and prognosis depends upon the site and extent of the disease. While in patients with localized disease the 5-year survival rate is approximately 65%, patients with advanced disease this figure drops to 36% (Godwin et al., 1975). Female gender and young age at diagnosis are associated with a better prognosis. Presence of metastases, high CgA level, and high proliferation index (Ki-67) are indicators of a poor outcome. Once, carcinoid heart disease was a troublesome complication and a cause of early death. With modern diagnostic and therapeutic technics this is rarely seen today. Development of a secondary malignancy, namely an adenocarcinoma of the large intestine, is another cause of reduced survival in these patients (Godwin et al., 1975). Whether combined adenocarcinoma and carcinoid tumors are a composite tumor or collision tumors has been debated (Yamashina & Flinner, 1985).

11. Conclusion

Neuroendocrine tumors continue to evolve with regard to diagnosis, classification epidemiology and treatment possibilities. They also provide a challenging source of testing novel drugs as their molecular targets have now started to be recognized.

12. References

Adamson AK, Grahame-Smith DG, Peart WS, & Starr M. (1969). Pharmacological blockade of carcinoid flushing provoked by catecholamines and alcohol. *Lancet* 1969;2:293.

Ahlman H, Kolby L, & Lundell L, et al., (1994). Clinical management of gastric carcinoid tumors. *Digestion* 1994;55(Suppl 3):77-85.

Anthony L, Vinik, AI. Pancreas. (2011). Evaluating the Characteristics and the Management of Patients With Neuroendocrine Tumors Receiving Octreotide LAR During a 6-Year Period. *Pancreas.* 40(7):987-994, October 2011. doi: 10.1097/MPA.0b013e31821f66b4)

Bajetta E, Rimassa L, & Carnaghi C, et al., (1998). 5-Fluorouracil, dacarbazine, and epirubicin in the treatment of patients with neuroendocrine tumors. *Cancer* 1998;83:372-378.

Bilimoria KY, Bentrem DJ, Wayne JD, Ko CY, Bennett CL, & Talamonti MS. (2009). Small bowel cancer in the United States: changes in epidemiology, treatment, and survival over the last 20 years. *Ann Surg.* 2009 Jan;249(1):63-71

Bosman FT, Carneiro F, Hruban RH, Theise ND (2010). *WHO classification of tumors of the digestive system*. Lyon, France: IARC Press; 2010.

Burke AP, Thomas RM, Elsayed AM, & Sobin LH. (1997). Carcinoids of the jejunum and ileum: an immunohistochemical and clinicopathologic study of 167 cases. *Cancer* 1997;79:1086-1093.

Buscail L, Esteve JP, & Saint-Laurent, et al., (1995). Inhibition of cell proliferation by the somatostatin analogue RC-160 is mediated by somatostatin receptor subtypes SSTR2 and SSTR5 through different mechanisms. *N Proc Natl Acad Sci USA* 1995;92:1580-1584.

Caldarola Vt, Jackman Rj, Moertel Cg, & Dockerty Mb. (1964). Carcinoid tumors of the rectum. *Am J Surg.* 1964;107:844-849.

Capella C, Heitz PU, Hofler H, Solcia E, & Kloppel G. (1995). Revised classification of neuroendocrine tumours of the lung, pancreas and gut. *Virchows Arch* 1995;425:547-560

Cattaneo MG, Amoroso D, & Gussoni G, et al., (1996). A somatostatin analogue inhibits MAP kinase activation and cell proliferation in human neuroblastoma and in human small cell lung carcinoma cell lines. *FEBS Lett* 1996;397:164-168.

Cordelier P, Esteve JP, & Bousquet C, et al., (1997). Characterization of the antiproliferative signal mediated by the somatostatin receptor subtype sst5. *Proc Natl Acad Sci USA* 1997;94:9343-9348.

Connolly HM, Nishimura RA, Smith HC, Pellikka PA, Mullany CJ, & Kvols LK. (1995). Outcome of cardiac surgery for carcinoid heart disease. *J Am Coll Cardiol* 1995;25:410-416.

Di Bartolomeo M, Bajetta E, & Bochicchio AM, et al., (1995). A phase II trial of dacarbazine, fluorouracil and epirubicin in patients with neuroendocrine tumours. A study by the Italian Trials in Medical Oncology (I.T.M.O.) Group. *Ann Oncol* 1995;6:77-79.

Dogan H. & Hot I. (2010). Contributions of Siegfried Oberndorfer to pathology and evolution of carcinoid. *Pol J Pathol.* 2010;61(1):49-53.

Doherty, GM. (2011). Neuroendocrine (carcinoid) tumors and the carcinoid syndrome, In: *Cancer Principles & Practice of Oncology*, DeVita, Jr. VT, Lawrence T, Rosenberg SA, pp. (1503-1515), Wolters Kluwer, Lippincott Williams & Wilkins, ISBN 978-1-4511-1813-1, Philadelphia

Dousset B, Saint-Marc O, Pitre J, Soubrane O, Houssin D, & Chapuis Y. (1996). Metastatic neuroendocrine tumors: medical treatment, surgical resection, or liver transplantation. *World J Surg* 1996;20:908-915.

Eriksson B, Arnberg H, Oberg K, Hellman U, Lundqvist G, Wernstedt C, Wilander E. (1990). *Acta Endocrinol (Copenh).* A polyclonal antiserum against chromogranin A and B--a new sensitive marker for neuroendocrine tumours. 1990:;122: 145-55.

Feldman JM & O'Dorisio TM (1986). Role of neuropeptides and serotonin in the diagnosis of carcinoid tumors. *Am J Med.* 1986: 81 (6B): 41-8.

Godwin JD 2nd. (1975). Carcinoid tumors. An analysis of 2,837 cases. *Cancer* 1975;36:560-569.

Goede AC, Caplin ME, & Winslet MC. (2003). Carcinoid tumour of the appendix. *Br J Surg* 2003; 90:1317-1322.

Gough DB, Thompson GB, & Crotty TB, et al., (1994). Diverse clinical and pathologic features of gastric carcinoid and the relevance of hypergastrinemia. *World J Surg* 1994;18:473-479.

Harpole DH Jr, Feldman JM, Buchanan S, Young WG, & Wolfe WG. (1992). Bronchial carcinoid tumors: a retrospective analysis of 126 patients. *Ann Thorac Surg* 1992;54:50-54.

Hoefnagel CA, den Hartog Jager FC, & Taal BG, et al., (1987). The role of I-131-MIBG in the diagnosis and therapy of carcinoids. *Eur J Nucl Med* 1987;13:187-191.

Imam H, Eriksson B, & Lukinius A, et al., (1997). Induction of apoptosis in neuroendocrine tumors of the digestive system during treatment with somatostatin analogs. *Acta Oncol.* 1997;36:607-614.

Jemore AB, Ray JE, & Gathright JB et al., (1992). Rectal carcinoids: the most frequent carcinoid tumour. *Dis Colon Rectum* 1992;35:717-725.

Kema IP, de Vries EG, & Muskiet FA. (2000). Clinical chemistry of serotonin and metabolites. *J Chromatogr B Biomed Sci Appl* 2000;747:33-48.

Kaplan B, Stevens CW, Allen P, Liao Z, & Komaki R. (2003). Outcomes and patterns of failure in bronchial carcinoid tumors. *Int J Radiat Oncol Biol Phys* 2003;55:125-131.

Kimmig BN. (1994). Radiotherapy for gastroenteropancreatic neuroendocrine tumors. *Ann N Y Acad Sci* 1994;733:488-495.

Klöppel G, Dege K, Remmele W, Kapran Y, Tuzlali S, Modlin IM. (2007). Siegfried Oberndorfer: a tribute to his work and life between Munich, Kiel, Geneva, and Istanbul. *Virchows Arch.* 2007 Aug;451 Suppl 1:S3-7. Epub 2007 Aug 8. Review

Kubota A, Yamada Y, & Kagimoto S, et al., (1994). Identification of somatostatin receptor subtypes and an implication for the efficacy of somatostatin analogue SMS 201-995 in treatment of human endocrine tumors. *J Clin Invest* 1994;93:1321-1325.

Kvols LK, Moertel CG, O'Connell MJ, Schutt AJ, Rubin J, & Hahn RG. (1986). Treatment of the malignant carcinoid syndrome: evaluation of a long-acting somatostatin analogue. *N Engl J Med* 1986;315:663-666.

Le Treut YP, Delpero JR, & Dousset B, et al., (1997). Results of liver transplantation in the treatment of metastatic neuroendocrine tumors: a 31-case French multicentric report. *Ann Surg* 1997;225:355-364.

Lubarsch O. (1888). Ueber den primaren Krebs des Ileum, nebst Bemerkungen u'ber das gleichzeitige Vorkommen von Krebs und Tuberkolose. *Virchows Arch* 1888;111:280-317.

Lundin L, Norheim I, Landelius J, Oberg K, Theodorsson-Norheim E. (1988). Carcinoid heart disease: relationship of circulating vasoactive substances to ultrasound-detectable cardiac abnormalities. *Circulation.* 1988 Feb;77(2):264-9.

Lundqvist M, & Wilander E. (1986). Subepithelial neuroendocrine cells and carcinoid tumours of the human small intestine and appendix: a comparative immunohistochemical study with regard to serotonin, neuron-specific enolase and S-100 protein reactivity. *J Pathol* 1986; 148:141-147

Maggard MA, O'Connell JB, & Ko CY. (2004). Updated population-based review of carcinoid tumors. *Ann Surg*, 2004;240:117-122.

Matsui K, Iwase T, & Kitagawa M. (1993). Small, polypoid-appearing carcinoid tumors of the rectum: clinicopathologic study of 16 cases and effectiveness of endoscopic treatment. *Am J Gastroenterol* 1993;88:1949-1953.

McEntee GP, Nagorney DM, Kvols LK, Moertel CG, & Grant CS. (1990). Cytoreductive hepatic surgery for neuroendocrine tumors. *Surgery* 1990;108:1091-1096.

Menda Y, & Kahn D. (2002). Somatostatin receptor imaging of non-small cell lung cancer with 99mTc depreotide. *Semin Nucl Med* 2002;32:92-96.

Modlin IM, & Sandor A. (1997). An analysis of 8305 cases of carcinoid tumors. *Cancer,* 1997;79:813-829.

Modlin IM, Lye KD, & Kidd M. (2003). A 5-decade analysis of 13,715 carcinoid tumors. *Cancer* 2003;97:934-959.

Moertel CG, Sauer WG, Dockerty MB, & Baggenstoss AH. (1961). Life history of the carcinoid tumor of the small intestine. *Cancer* 1961;14:901-912.

Moertel CG, Dockerty MB, & Judd ES. (1968). Carcinoid tumors of the vermiform appendix. *Cancer* 1968;21:270-278.

Moertel CG, Weiland LH, Nagorney DM, & Dockerty MB. (1987). Carcinoid tumor of the appendix: treatment and prognosis. *N Engl J Med* 1987;317:1699-1701.

Moertel CG, Kvols LK, & O'Connell MJ, et al., (1991). Treatment of neuroendocrine carcinomas with combined etoposide and cisplatin. Evidence of major therapeutic activity in the anaplastic variants of these neoplasms. *Cancer* 1991;68:227-232.

Moses RE, Frank BB, Leavitt M, & Miller R. (1986).The syndrome of type A chronic atrophic gastritis, pernicious anemia, and multiple gastric carcinoids. *J Clin Gastroenterol* 1986;8:61-65.

Nassar AA, Jaroszewski DE, Helmers RA, Colby TV, Patel BM, Mookadam F. (2011) Diffuse idiopathic pulmonary neuroendocrine cell hyperplasia: a systematic overview. *Am J Respir Crit Care Med.* 2011 Jul 1;184(1):8-16. Epub 2011 Mar 25

Nessi R, Basso Ricci P, Basso Ricci S, Bosco M, Blanc M, & Uslenghi C. (1991). Bronchial carcinoid tumors: radiologic observations in 49 cases. *J Thorac Imaging* 1991;6:47-53.

Norheim I, Oberg K, Theodorsson-Norheim E, Lindgren PG, Lundqvist G, Magnusson A, Wide L, & Wilander E. (1987). Malignant carcinoid tumors. An analysis of 103 patients with regard to tumor localization, hormone production, and survival. *Ann Surg* 1987;206:115-125.

Oberg K, Norheim I, & Lind E, et al., (1986). Treatment of malignant carcinoid tumors with human leukocyte interferon: long-term results. *Cancer Treat Rep* 1986;70:1297-1304.

Oberndorfer S. (1907). Karcinoide Tumoren des Dunndarms. *Frankfurt II Pathol* 1907;1:1426-1429.

O'Dorisio TM, Krutzik SR, Woltering EA, Lindholm E, Joseph S, Gandolfi AE, Wang YZ, Boudreaux JP, Vinik AI, Go VL, Howe JR, Halfdanarson T, O'Dorisio MS, Mamikunian G. (2010). Development of a highly sensitive and specific carboxy-terminal human pancreastatin assay to monitor neuroendocrine tumor behavior. *Pancreas.* 2010 Jul;39(5):611-6.

Orlefors H, Sundin A, Ahlstrom H, Bjurling P, Bergstrom M, Lilja A, Langstrom B, Oberg K, & Eriksson B. (1998). Positron emission tomography with 5-hydroxytryprophan in neuroendocrine tumors. *J Clin Oncol* 1998;16:2534-2541.

Que FG, Nagorney DM, Batts KP, Linz LJ, & Kvols LK. (1995). Hepatic resection for metastatic neuroendocrine carcinomas. *Am J Surg* 1995;169:36-43.

Paties C, Zangrandi A, Vassallo G, Rindi G, Solcia E. (1991). Multidirectional carcinoma of the thymus with neuroendocrine and sarcomatoid components and carcinoid syndrome. *Pathol Res Pract.* 1991 Mar;187(2-3):170-7.

Raymond E, Dahan L, Raoul JL, Bang YJ, Borbath I, Lombard-Bohas C, Valle J, Metrakos P, Smith D, Vinik A, Chen JS, Hörsch D, Hammel P, Wiedenmann B, Van Cutsem E, Patyna S, Lu DR, Blanckmeister C, Chao R, Ruszniewski P. (2011). Sunitinib malate for the treatment of pancreatic neuroendocrine tumors. N Engl J Med. 2011 Feb 10;364(6):501-13. Erratum in: N Engl J Med. 2011 Mar 17;364(11):1082.

Rindi G, Luinetti O, Cornaggia M, Capella C, & Solcia E. (1993). Three subtypes of gastric argyrophil carcinoid and the gastric neuroendocrine carcinoma: a clinicopathologic study. *Gastroenterology* 1993;104:994-1006.

Robiolio PA, Rigolin VH, & Harrison JK, et al., (1995). Predictors of outcome of tricuspid valve replacement in carcinoid heart disease. *Am J Cardiol* 1995;75:485-488.

Rosenberg JM, & Welch JP. (1985). Carcinoid tumors of the colon: a study of 72 patients. *Am J Surg* 1985;149:775-779.

Safford SD, Coleman RE, Gockerman JP, Moore J, Feldman J, Onaitis MW, Tyler DS, & Olson JA Jr. (2004). Iodine-131 metaiodobenzylguanidine treatment for metastatic carcinoid. Results in 98 patients. Cancer 2004;101:1987-1993.

Scarpignato C, & Pelosini I. (2001). Somatostatin analogs for cancer treatment and diagnosis: an overview. *Chemotherapy* 2001;47(Suppl 2):1-29.

Schott, M; Klöppel, G; Raffel, A; Saleh, A; Knoefel, W T; Scherbaum, WA. (2011). Neuroendocrine Neoplasms of the Gastrointestinal Tract. *Dtsch Arztebl Int* 2011; 108(18): 305-12

Schupak KD, & Wallner KE. (1991). The role of radiation therapy in the treatment of locally unresectable or metastatic carcinoid tumors. *Int J Radiat Oncol Biol Phys* 1991;20:489-495.

Shaw PA. (1990). Carcinoid tumours of the appendix are different. J Pathol 1990;612:189-190.

Sjoblom SM, Sipponen P, & Jarvinen H. (1993). Gastroscopic follow-up of pernicious anaemia patients. Gut 1993;34:28-32.

Smith RA. (1969). Bronchial carcinoid tumours. Thorax 1969;24:43-50.

Strosberg JR, Fine RL, Choi J, Nasir A, Coppola D, Chen DT, Helm J, Kvols L. (2011). First-line chemotherapy with capecitabine and temozolomide in patients with metastatic pancreatic endocrine carcinomas. Cancer. 2011; Jan 15;117(2):268-75. doi: 10.1002/cncr.25425. Epub 2010 Sep 7.

Sundin A, Eriksson B, Bergstrom M, Langstrom B, Oberg K, & Orlefors H. (2004). PET in the diagnosis of neuroendocrine tumors. *Ann N Y Acad Sci* 2004;1014:246-257.

Sutton R, Doran HE, & Williams EM, et al., (2003). Surgery for midgut carcinoid. *Endocr Relat Cancer* 2003; 10:469-481.

Thompson GB, van Heerden JA, Martin JK Jr, Schutt AJ, Ilstrup DM, & Carney JA. (1985). Carcinoid tumors of the gastrointestinal tract: presentation, management, and prognosis. Surgery. 1985;98:1054-63.

Thorson A, Biorck G, & Bjorkman G, Waldenstrom J. (1954). Malignant carcinoid of the small intestine with metastases to the liver, valvular disease of the right side of the heart (pulmonary stenosis and tricuspid regurgitation without septal defects), peripheral vasomotor symptoms, bronchoconstriction, and an unusual type of cyanosis; a clinical and pathologic syndrome. *Am Heart J* 1954;47:795-817.

Taal BG, Hoefnagel CA, & Valdes Olmos RA, et al., (1996). Palliative effect of metaiodobenzylguanidine in metastatic carcinoid tumors. J Clin Oncol 1996;14:1829-1838.

Vinik A. (January 28, 2008). Carcinoid Tumors, In: *Endotext,* October 30, 2011, Available from: http://www.endotext.org/guthormones/guthormone2/guthormoneframe2.htm

Waldherr C, Pless M, Maecke HR, Haldemann A, & Mueller-Brand J. (2001). The clinical value of [90Y-DOTA]-D-Phe1-Tyr3-octreotide (90Y-DOTATOC) in the treatment of neuroendocrine tumours: a clinical phase II study. *Ann Oncol* 2001;12:941-945.

Williams ED, & Sandler M. (1963). The classification of carcinoid tumours. *Lancet* 1963;1:238-239.

Yamashina M & Flinner RA. (1985). Concurrent occurrence of adenocarcinoma and carcinoid tumour in the stomach: A composite tumour or collision tumors? Am J *Clin Pathol* 1985;83:233-6.

Yao JC, Phan A, Hoff PM, Chen NX, Charnsangavej C, Yeung SC, Hess K, Ng C, Abbruzzese JC, & Ajani JA. (2008) Targeting vascular endothelial growth factor in advanced carcinoid tumor: a random assignment phase II study of depot octreotide with bevacizumab and pegylated interferon alpha-2b. *J Clin Oncol.* Vol.26, 2008 Mar 10; 26(8):1316-23.

Yao JC, Hassan M, Phan A, Dagohoy C, Leary C, Mares JE, Abdalla EK, Fleming JB, Vauthey JN, Rashid A, Evans DB. (2008). One hundred years after "carcinoid": epidemiology of and prognostic factors for neuroendocrine tumors in 35,825 cases in the United States. *J Clin Oncol.* 2008 Jun 20;26(18):3063-72

Yao JC, Shah MH, Ito T, Bohas CL, Wolin EM, Van Cutsem E, Hobday TJ, Okusaka T, Capdevila J, de Vries EG, Tomassetti P, Pavel ME, Hoosen S, Haas T, Lincy J, Lebwohl D, Öberg K; RAD001 in Advanced Neuroendocrine Tumors, Third Trial (RADIANT-3) Study Group. (2011). Everolimus for advanced pancreatic neuroendocrine tumors. *N Engl J Med.* 2011 Feb 10;364(6):514-23.

Yildiz O, Ozguroglu M (2006). Carcinoid tumors, In:*Neuroendocrine Tumors of Gastroenteropanceatic System,* Suayip Yalcin, Huseyin Abali, pp. (117-135), Form Reklam Hizmetleri, ISBN:975-00787-0-5, Ankara

Yildiz O, Ozguroglu M, Yanmaz T, Turna H, Serdengecti S, Dogusoy G. (2010) Gastroenteropancreatic neuroendocrine tumors: 10-year experience in a single center. *Med Oncol.* 2010 Dec;27(4):1050-6. Epub 2009 Nov 3.

Zar N, Garmo H, Holmberg L, Rastad J, & Hellman P. (2004). Long-term Survival of Patients with Small Intestinal Carcinoid Tumors. *World J Surg* 2004;28:1163-1168.